DELETED

Cocaine

Cocaine

An In-Depth Look at the Facts, Science, History and Future of the World's Most Addictive Drug

JOHN C. FLYNN

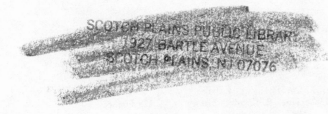
A Citadel Press Book
Published by Carol Publishing Group

Carol Publishing Group Edition - 1993

Copyright © 1991 by John C. Flynn

A Citadel Press Book
Published by Carol Publishing Group
Citadel Press is a registered trademark of Carol Communications, Inc.

Editorial Offices: 600 Madison Avenue, New York, NY 10022
Sales & Distribution Offices: 120 Enterprise Avenue, Secaucus, NJ 07094
In Canada: Canadian Manda Group, P.O. Box 920, Station U, Toronto,
Ontario, M8Z 5P9, Canada

Queries regarding rights and permissions should be addressed to:
Carol Publishing Group, 600 Madison Avenue, New York, NY 10022

Lyrics from "I Get a Kick Out of You" by Cole Porter © 1934
Warner Bros. Inc. (Renewed) All Rights Reserved. Used by permission.

Manufactured in the United States of America
ISBN 0-8065-1432-9

10 9 8 7 6 5 4 3 2 1

Carol Publishing Group books are available at special discounts
for bulk purchases, for sales promotions, fund raising, or
educational purposes. Special editions can also be created to
specifications. For details contact: Special Sales Department,
Carol Publishing Group, 120 Enterprise Ave., Secaucus, NJ 07094

Library of Congress Cataloging-in-Publication Data

Flynn, John C.
        Cocaine : an in-depth look at the facts, science, history, and
    future of the world's most addictive drug/ by John C. Flynn.
            p.   cm.
        "A Citadel Press book."
        Includes index.
        1. Cocaine. 2. Cocaine habit. I. Title.
        [DNLM: 1. Cocaine. 2. Cocaine--history. QV 113 F648c]
    QP801.C68F48   1991
        616.86'47--dc20
    DNLM/DLC   91-201
        for Library of Congress   CIP

To my wife,
Elli

Contents

Preface xi

1. Helen's Story, or "How Did I Get Into This Mess?" 1

2. A Brief History of a Most Unusual Drug 17

3. The Different Faces of Paradise 32

4. What It's Like to "Do Cocaine" 47

5. Pleasure, Pleasure and More Pleasure: Cocaine, the Brain
   and Addiction 68

6. Unlocking the Pleasure Centers: How the Key Works 84

7. How Bad Is It? The Scope of the Cocaine Problem 104

8. How Bad Can It Get? What Lies Beyond Cocaine? 121

9. Rethinking the Future Beyond Cocaine 144

   Index 163

Acknowledgments

I would like to express my gratitude to several people who have helped and encouraged me in the writing of this book. My good friend, academic colleague and fellow writer, Dr. Lewis M. Barker, read early versions of the manuscript and provided many useful comments and suggestions. My editor at Birch Lane Press, Bruce Shostak, improved the manuscript with his expert touch. Ruth Wreschner, my agent, deserves special thanks for her work in my behalf. Finally, my wife, Dr. Eleanor R. Flynn, provided the encouragement and support that made writing the book possible. She also, in her many readings of early drafts, kept the reader's viewpoint in front of me, with her insistent demands for clear and straightforward prose.

Any errors of fact in the book are, of course, mine.

JOHN C. FLYNN

Preface

Americans feel besieged by drugs. They rank drug abuse and the traffic in illegal substances among the most pressing domestic problems facing the nation. They believe the problem extends beyond our borders as well. With the sudden end of the cold war, many Americans are inclined to the view that halting the flow of cocaine into the United States is one of the more pressing of our foreign policy problems. This concern with drugs is mirrored in the media, where news reports, feature articles and special programing address the issues on a daily basis. Politicians, too, respond to this concern. Rare is the seeker of public office today who does not feel compelled to make clear his position on the drug problem.

What many of us do not realize, however, is that the drug problem is not entirely new. It did not begin suddenly a decade ago with the widespread use of cocaine. It did not begin in the 1960s, with marijuana-smoking, LSD-dropping flower children. The illegal use of mind-altering substances is a lot older than that. The *legal* use of such substances in our society is even older. Our recreational drug use (that is, the use of drugs for the express purpose of altering normal mental states, as opposed to their medical or self-prescribed use in treating illness) may be more widespread now, but it is not new. We have been using drugs, legally and illegally, for precisely these purposes for many years.

We are not alone in this. The use of drugs to alter mental states, to change the way we feel about ourselves and the world around us, transcends our time and place. It is common in many societies other than our own and has occurred throughout history. References to what is probably the opium poppy are found in Sumerian tablets dating to 3000 B.C. The drugs may differ from time to time and from place to place, but the effect sought remains the same.

Why, then, are we bedeviled in 1991 with a cocaine problem that seems to have spiraled out of control? If we have had so much experience with mind-altering substances, why do we not do a better job of dealing with them? Why, in addition to cocaine, do heroin, marijuana, LSD, PCP and amphetamines continue to torment us, in spite of many years of our best efforts to control their use? I suggest in this book that we have done such a poor job because we have never understood the nature of the problem. I suggest, moreover, that unless we begin soon to reexamine the problem, progress in the struggle to reduce the damage wrought by drugs will continue to elude us. In fact, failure to carry out such a reassessment *now* may guarantee that drug problems of the future will be more severe than they are today.

There is an urgent need for a new understanding of drug use and drug abuse. Narcotics like heroin are still with us. They constitute, if anything, a bigger problem than they did in 1914 when the first major federal legislation was enacted to regulate them. Additional drugs have appeared on the scene since then—LSD, marijuana, PCP, amphetamines and inhalants, to mention a few. As they assumed prominence among drug abusers, strenuous efforts were made to control their use. These drugs, too, are still with us. Like the narcotics, they continue to resist our best efforts to curb their use.

It is the reappearance of cocaine, however, in epidemic proportions, that forces us to rethink the problems of drug abuse. Note that I speak of a *reappearance* of cocaine. This drug was widely used earlier in our history, notably in the late nineteenth and early twentieth centuries. For this reason it was included as a drug to be regulated by federal legislation in 1914. The current blizzard of cocaine testifies loudly that we have yet to understand why our efforts to curtail its use have failed.

The resurgence of cocaine presents us with an imperative. It suggests that we had better come to an improved understanding of the nature of drug use and drug abuse, and we had better do it *now*. We must gain a clearer insight into the lure that some chemical compounds have for so many people. For as pharmacologists and neuroscientists well know, the future is very likely to see the emergence of drugs that are even more beguiling, even more addicting than cocaine. Unless we reach an improved understanding of the reasons why such drugs are irresistible to so many people, an understanding that finds expression in public policy, it is highly likely that we will experience drug problems in the future that dwarf those facing us today.

Cocaine has forced a reexamination of our thinking because, in important respects, cocaine is different than most of the other drugs that trouble us. Of paramount importance is that cocaine is different in the way it affects the brain. Cocaine acts on the brain cells responsible for our ability to experience pleasure. Other drugs, like heroin, are also capable of stimulating pleasure circuits in the brain. The fact that they lead to feelings of pleasure is one reason they are abused. Cocaine, however, stimulates these brain areas more directly than other drugs, which is why, in its various forms, it is used so compulsively.

It is only recently that science has begun to understand these differences. This new understanding demands that we reevaluate much of our thinking about the use and abuse of drugs. It suggests that we make a fundamental error in classifying very different drugs, drugs that act differently in the brain, under the common heading of *drugs of abuse*. The error is fundamental because it usually leads inexorably to the conclusion that all such drugs can be dealt with in the same way, using the same policies, simply because we have decreed that they are all drugs of abuse. This error lies at the root of our meager success in dealing with the recent onslaught of cocaine.

More generally, cocaine provides us with another imperative. It is the imperative to think critically about drugs and their use and abuse in our society. This imperative to think requires that we ask more questions about drugs than we have been inclined to ask. We must ask detailed questions about each drug individually, about how it acts in specific ways in the human brain. We must find out all we can about each drug. When this is done, we will find that we do not have a single drug problem which demands a single solution. We will see that we have different problems with different drugs, which, in all probability, will require a variety of solutions.

This book attempts to view cocaine in this light. It takes cocaine as a case study of a highly addictive drug. Its origins and chemical nature are examined. Its use and abuse throughout history are detailed. The effects of the drug on various organ systems of the body are explored, as are the subjective responses of people experiencing these effects. Most important, a careful inquiry is conducted into the action of the drug in the human brain. In that context it will be seen that cocaine is a chemical key that unlocks and activates brain circuits that make the experience of pleasure possible, circuits that have evolved in animals because they are fundamental to the survival of the individual and the species.

The starting point of this journey is the story of a young woman, Helen, whose cocaine use led to a severe crisis in her life. She and her boyfriend, Charley, are composite personalities. They have been drawn to illustrate common themes in one's introduction to cocaine, its continued use and the havoc it can bring about in individual lives. Some readers may find in Helen and Charley echoes of their own experience. It is my hope that all readers find in the book an enhanced understanding of the drug problem in America. I hope, also, that they are stimulated to ask new questions about how to solve it.

Cocaine

Chapter 1

Helen's Story, or "How Did I Get Into This Mess?"

Let me tell you about Helen.

You'd like her. Everybody does. She's warm, outgoing and easy to know, the kind of person who makes friends readily. Her effortless smile and infectious laugh suggest an openness that draws people to her. She is a bright, ambitious, hardworking, young professional whose career is definitely upward bound.

When she was brought into the emergency room of Community General Hospital at 11:00 P.M., she looked like someone who had just come face to face with some unspeakable evil. Her face was a mask of terror. Bent over slightly from the waist, her shoulders hunched up around her ears, she sat rigidly on the edge of the examination table. Her eyebrows were arched upward into her forehead and her lower jaw was held downward and to the rear. This contortion of her facial muscles had stretched her skin taut over the bony structure beneath. Her eyes darted rapidly back and forth at the small cluster of people surrounding her. The undeniable fear etched into her face and the vacant quality of her gaze suggested that her mind was not processing what her eyes were seeing. Indeed, the questions being put to Helen by the people around her were of little importance compared to the chaos that was exploding inside her head.

"Helen." White Coat was speaking. "Helen, I'm Doctor Walsh. Can you hear me? Helen, can you tell me what the trouble is?"

Helen knew that White Coat was speaking to her. She was even vaguely aware that he might be able to help. That possibility of help sent a surge of hope, brief but recognizable, into the awful confusion and disorder that reigned in her mind. She tried to concentrate on the voice. She knew it belonged to White Coat, but it didn't seem to be coming from White Coat. She tried hard to locate it, to fix it rigidly in space—that would be something to hold on to. She slowly scanned the room, her eyes darting furtively. But she couldn't find the voice. It seemed to be coming from far away, like a puff of air whose effect is constantly diminished as it proceeds outward from its source.

Finally, it didn't seem very significant. Locating the voice required an inordinate amount of concentration, more than she could muster, and the whole process was made more difficult by the rushing sound of wind in her head. The blowing and whistling noises, varying suddenly and without warning in amplitude and pitch, sprang out of a constant, dull background roar to assault her with wave after wave of uncontrollable fury. And flashing lights, like the rushing wind, were creating a disturbance inside her head. They had started as a minor annoyance that distracted her and made concentration difficult; now they were terrifying. They popped and crackled in a multicolored display of reds, blues, purples, oranges and the brightest, most dazzling bolts of lightning she had ever seen. So dazzling were they that she thought they might blind her. Sometimes the lights seemed to explode out of her head and into the room, where they illuminated the entire scene with shafts of ricocheting light. At other times they raced toward her, into the very interior of her brain, threatening to explode her head into a thousand pieces.

"Stop the lights!" she screamed, pounding on her temples with her fists. "Please! Please, stop the lights!"

"Helen." It was White Coat again, speaking more urgently now and holding each of her hands in order to restrain her from hitting herself again. "Helen," he said more firmly now, "tell me what the lights are like."

Without warning, Helen's body straightened on the edge of the table, her eyes rolled back in their sockets, she expelled air forcefully from her lungs in a kind of muted cry, and before anyone could prevent it, she catapulted off the examination table and crashed to the floor, where she lay thrashing in a paroxysm of violent contractions.

"Grand mal! Grand mal!"

"Seizure!"

"Somebody get her tongue!"

Helen was not able to hear these cries of the emergency room personnel. The convulsion had rendered her unconscious. The violent and chaotic firestorm in her brain, the synchronous discharge of millions of brain cells running riot, had overwhelmed her awareness of the world around her. Mercifully, she would have no memory of lying, as she now was, on the cold, tile floor, her body trembling with the residual muscular tremors that marked the effort of her brain to reestablish some sense of normal control over its own function.

It would take some time for her brain to complete this process. The task facing that complex organ was to regain its control over Helen's life. The restorative work would be done over a period of days. It would begin with the relatively easy parts of the job. Control would be regained first over the movement of large muscle groups, those muscles which had spiraled out of control to pitch her onto the floor and wrack her body with the spastic contractions of a grand mal seizure. This first step in the restorative process had begun even while Helen was trembling on the hospital floor. The major convulsions were over. The residual tremors and muted jerkings were evidence that the brain was now in the process of bringing the more finely tuned smaller muscles back under control.

Memory is a more delicate manner. It would take more time for Helen's brain to complete the exquisitely subtle adjustments that transform events into memories, thus making a continuity of existence possible. And this work would never be quite complete. Some damage would not be repairable. There would always be holes in Helen's memory. And although the presence of these gaps would nag at her in the weeks to come, they held an element of mercy. For just as she would have no memory of the convulsion, neither would she have a clear recollection of the ensuing train of diagnostic and treatment procedures that Dr. Walsh orchestrated during the next phase of her emergency room ordeal. She would not remember being lifted from the floor and being flopped unceremoniously on the examination table. She would not remember strong fingers trying to pry her jaws apart, holding her down and momentarily struggling at cross-purposes with those other hands that were trying to get her back on the table. She would have no memory of the needle pricks and the binding of the medical tape as intravenous lines were started to infuse her body with the various drugs and medications that would be necessary to treat her. There would be no memory of the padded tongue depressor being jammed between her teeth. (It was too late for that precaution, anyway; she had already severely bitten her tongue. Her teeth had cut completely through it on the right side. The painful healing of the wound would be a constant reminder in the days to come that something awful had happened to her this evening.)

Then, over the next few days, as the restorative process continued, her memory for ongoing events would improve. She would begin to recognize with certainty that she was in the hospital at about the same time that she confronted the horror of not having any recollection of how or why she was there. Gradually, short memory spans would link discrete events and anchor them in her awareness, eventually forming them into a continuous time along which she could once again chart her existence. As her memory improved, the hospital events that she could remember would stand out starkly in her mind. They would be separated by an unbridgeable gap from the fragmentary memories that the convulsion had left intact of the events that had led up to her hospitalization.

Dr. Walsh was curious to know what those events might have been. The scene in the emergency room had developed so quickly that he had received only very sketchy reports from the admissions people. When things had calmed down a bit, he began to fill in some of the gaps. After he had satisfied himself that Helen was stabilized and out of danger, he turned to the admission sheet containing the report of the paramedics who had brought her to the hospital. He looked through the report for key words and phrases that would aid in his diagnosis.

From the admission data he learned that the paramedics had been called to a home in an affluent section of town in response to a report that an individual there was acting "sort of hysterical and out of control." It was evident to the paramedics that a party was, or had been, in progress. The kitchen and living room were strewn with empty beer bottles and half-full glasses of wine. There was the unmistakable smell of marijuana in the air. On a low coffee table in the living room was a small mirror and several razor blades. There were traces of a white powder scattered over the surface of the mirror. The number of glasses in evidence suggested that some people must have left before the paramedics arrived. Still other people were hurriedly leaving as the ambulance pulled into the driveway. Five people other than Helen were still in the house. All of them seemed to be stoned and not overly concerned with the medics' attempts to find out who needed assistance.

The paramedics had found Helen sitting alone on the floor in a corner of the kitchen. Her legs were pulled up under her chin and her arms were wrapped tightly around her knees. A miniature ceramic pipe lay at her feet. Her eyes darted rapidly back and forth around the room, never seeming to focus on anything in particular. They did not focus on the paramedics as they attempted to question her. She was agitated and appeared to be fearful. She responded to their questions only obliquely, seeming to be much more interested in whatever it was that her eyes were following around the room. She complained of head pain and of being bothered by flashing lights. She was too agitated and disoriented to comply with their request that she lie down on the gurney. The two paramedics half carried her between them to the ambulance and took her directly to the hospital emergency room.

Walsh knew the rest. His own examination, begun once the convulsions had subsided, indicated that Helen was a young woman (her driver's license said that she was twenty-six years old), well dressed and well nourished. Upon admittance to the emergency room, her blood pressure was elevated to an alarming level, her pupils were dilated, she had a fever of 102 degrees, her heart rate was 125 beats per minute and the electrocardiogram (ECG) revealed irregular cardiac rhythms. Her skin was noticeably red, and she was sweating profusely. The nasal septum, the cartilage dividing the two nostrils, was perforated. She remained quite agitated and confused throughout the examination.

After about thirty minutes, most of Helen's physical symptoms had declined in severity. Her blood pressure had returned to near normal limits; the fever had declined to 100 degrees; her heart rate was down to 95 beats per minute; sweating had ceased; her pupils had returned to normal size. Helen's mental status showed gradual improvement during this period. She was considerably less agitated, although she remained quite confused and disoriented.

Dr. Walsh was fairly confident that he knew what had precipitated Helen's crisis. While a definitive diagnosis would have to wait until the completion of a history and the results of various laboratory tests, his tentative diagnosis was quite clear in his mind: his patient was suffering from a toxic reaction to cocaine.

Why Didn't Anybody Tell Me?

Helen didn't know what she was getting into. She had no idea when she began using cocaine that she could end up as a crisis case in the emergency room of a hospital. She did not use other drugs, not even marijuana—it made her sick. She drank alcohol on the weekends, but rarely drank to excess. Alcohol was, as she put it, "a way of mellowing out."

Certainly she had no inkling that the drug she tried so casually, at the urging of her friends, could have long-run consequences that were so different from the immediate feelings of pleasure that she experienced when she first tried it. Listen to her description, given several weeks following her release from the hospital, of that first exposure to cocaine.

"I was at a party with some new people and I was feeling pretty mellow and laid back. Charley, my fiancé, had already tried a hit. They kinda coaxed me and teased me, and Charley was telling me what a blast it was, so I went along. This friend of Charley's put a couple of lines on the table and showed me what to do. He told me that I should first rub a little coke on my gums with my finger. Then he gave me a rolled up dollar bill and showed me how to snort it up my nose. And I did.

"It was unbelievable. There's no other way to put it. I didn't know it was possible to feel so good! I mean, not in any specific way. Just good. The party had been going on for some time and I was pretty mellowed out. When I snorted the coke, nothing happened for a while, like for maybe three or four minutes. Then, it was like the whole world opened up to me. Everything seemed great. I felt kinda wired, but not in a bad way. Like, I just had a lot of energy. I felt like I could do anything I wanted to. All of the input that I was getting from the people in the room had a new kind of fascination to it. It was like my nerves had become more sensitive to what was happening and I was more responsive to all of it. It was a real turn-on."

At the time of this experience, Helen was a responsible, upwardly mobile young professional. She was dedicated to her career in computer applications in the business world. Her current position was that of a highly paid systems analyst. Charley, her fiancé, was a certified public accountant with a large firm. His future was as bright as hers. Helen had a new car that she traded every other year, a tastefully furnished apartment and a man that she deeply loved. She had no way of knowing what was to come.

What was to come was an increasing involvement with cocaine, an involvement that would jeopardize everything that she valued in her life. As this involvement intensified, she would see her job performance slip to the point of endangering her promising career. Her relationship with Charley would be strained to the breaking point. She would end up in the hospital with her life at risk.

The basic fact is that Helen, and Charley as well, came to like cocaine more than they ever would have imagined possible. Perhaps "like" is not a strong enough word to describe the attraction that they felt. They were drawn to it in a way that was new to them. Unlike drinking alcohol, which for them was merely one of many related activities that constituted a relaxing evening, cocaine soon became center stage, a star, the stand-out, one-of-a-kind activity that provided the whole reason for having the evening.

They began doing the drug at parties with friends. As the cocaine use increased, these parties would last all weekend. There was a lot of alcohol and plenty of cocaine. There was also sex. Cocaine seemed to make sex better, and during these marathon weekends when nobody slept, it made sex much more likely. Helen's recollection of those times tells the story.

"Jeeze, the whole thing is hard to believe. We didn't know what was happening. Neither of us.

"We really both got into the high. At first, Charley more than I did. . . . But, hey, I don't mean to lay it all off on Charley. It's as much my fault as his. But once we started concentrating on the drug, once it became our thing, a thing that we did by ourselves, not just at parties, then we were screwed. We couldn't turn it off.

"At first, a lot of the push did come from Charley ... but no way am I blaming him. I should have been able to handle it. But it became such a sexual turn-on for him that he didn't want to go out any more. He wanted to stay home a lot, get high and make love. There was a lot of that kind of stuff at the parties, you know, but we could never get into it. ... You know, swapping partners and all that stuff. So we stayed home more and more and did coke."

Helen found herself increasingly withdrawn from her relationships with friends. The world that she inhabited with Charley became progressively restricted. Just as their outside interests decreased, so did their interest in their work. They worked at their jobs during the day, each of them with mounting ineffectiveness, all the while looking forward to the evening when they could return home and do more cocaine. With hindsight, Helen was able to see the way the events unfolded.

"The damn drug took us away from other people and finally ended up by taking us away from each other. After a while the only thing that was important was cocaine. *We* didn't even count anymore.

"See ... what happens is that when you're doing enough coke the downside gets to be unbearable. So you do more. And more. And when you do enough of it, you get to the point that the only thing that matters, the only thing that can pick you up, the only thing that gives you any pleasure at all, is the goddam cocaine.

"It's unbelievable, in a way. We started out doing coke to get high and have fabulous sex. At least that kept us close, kept us holding on to each other. But toward the end we didn't even have sex anymore. It wasn't as good as the cocaine. All we wanted to do was stay high, and finally we didn't even care about what the other person was feeling, or what the other person was all about.

"We became like the proverbial ships that pass in the night. We floated by each other on a sea of cocaine. Each one of us was intent on steering his own course. We were aware of one another only to the extent of trying to avoid a collision in the dark."

Does Anybody Know What's Going On?

The fact that Helen was so ignorant of what lay in store for her represents one of the real ironies of the present day. *This is a drug-*

intoxicated culture that understands almost nothing about drugs. Drugs in the United States are dealt with mostly by catchwords and slogans: "addict," "dope-head," "just say no," "zero tolerance," "restrict supply," "reduce demand" and so on.

The trouble with catchwords and slogans is that they too often make very complicated problems seem simpler than they really are. Catchwords conceal the complexity of a problem under a superficial layer of apparent understanding. Helen's lack of knowledge of the possible consequences of her cocaine use is due, in large part, to her willingness to accept this kind of sloganeering as a substitute for knowledge.

Not that she didn't think that she had a lot of information. She ran with a hip crowd, a switched-on, get-it-while-you-can crowd. And they all "knew a lot about cocaine." What they knew was revealed in their conversation.

"Hey! This is a real mindblower!"

"If you're hung over, a little snort will fix you right up."

"Don't lick up the leavings with your tongue. It's bitter as hell. Better to rub it on your gums."

"When you have sex while you're on this stuff, it's like it's never gonna end."

Helen never took the time to inform herself about the drug that she so casually accepted from her friends. It did not occur to her to ask questions about what the drug did to her mind. She was even less inclined to wonder about how cocaine affected her brain in order to do these things to her mind. Furthermore, even if she had thought to ask such questions, it is unlikely that she would have found any answers close at hand. Certainly not from her fellow drug users. None of these people had any real information about cocaine. Their knowledge was concerned largely with the folklore of the drug, most of which had little to do with the descent into addiction that Helen experienced.

In a similar way, the dismal failure to stop the spread of destructive drug use in our society is due to our acceptance of catchwords, glib phrases and slogans. These have insulated most people from the realities of the cocaine problem in much the same way that Helen was isolated from knowledge about the drug, knowledge that could have prevented her destruction. Cocaine continues to be a scourge of contemporary life largely because society, from the top levels of government to the man in the street, has preferred slogans to information, and ignorance to knowledge.

There is nothing new about all of this. From the very beginning, the preference for slogans and glib phrases as a substitute for knowledge has been characteristic of our approach to "the drug problem" (another slogan!). We have dealt with heroin, marijuana, LSD, peyote, amphetamine, PCP, and a host of other drugs in just this way, and not very successfully, either. These drugs are still with us. They still take a frightening toll in our society. They continue to act as snares that trap thousands of our young people every year. Our approach to "the drug problem" has not rid society of the scourge of drugs. Rather, the scourge has become steadily worse.

In fact, the most dangerous of all of these glib phrases is "the drug problem." Because of it, we have been led to believe that all drugs are alike, that all drug abuse is alike. In the name of "the drug problem" we have been told that all drug abusers are alike. Once we have come to accept this simplistic view of the problem, it is easy to make us see what the solution is. We can solve "the drug problem" posed by cocaine in the same time-honored ways that we've used to solve "the drug problem" posed by heroin or marijuana or amphetamine or LSD or any other drug. The only thing we're *not* told is that these time-honored ways have never really solved *any* of these other drug problems.

Reality is much more complicated than the slogan-makers would have us believe. It is simply not true that all drugs are alike. One of the disastrous mistakes we have made is to assume that merely labeling something a "drug" conveys all the information that is needed in order to talk reasonably about that substance. The grouping of wildly different substances under the common heading of "drugs" or "drugs of abuse," and then assuming that, since they are all called by the same name, they all can be dealt with in the same way, is the single most important factor in our failure to control "the drug problem" in the United States.

The information, for example, that heroin, amphetamine, cocaine and alcohol are all drugs of abuse should *not* lead to the conclusion that no other information is needed in order to devise rational strategies for dealing with people who abuse them. Rather, the question should be asked up front: "Is it possible that important differences exist among these drugs of abuse, differences which suggest that the solutions applied to one of them may not apply to the others?"

The fact is that no two drugs are identical. It is also a fact that problems of abuse differ from drug to drug. Addiction to heroin is quite different in many important ways than addiction to alcohol. The differences are so great, in fact, that a physician would never try to treat them in the same way. If he were to treat a person addicted to alcohol in the same way that he treats an individual addicted to morphine, his alcohol-dependent patient would very likely die. Whereas withdrawal from morphine can be serious and most unpleasant, it is not potentially lethal. Withdrawal of the physiologically dependent person from alcohol, on the other hand, can be life-threatening. The morphine-dependent person can withdraw "cold turkey" and survive. An alcohol-dependent person should be hospitalized where he can be maintained on suitable medication and protected from dangerous seizures.

All of this can be said in another way. We don't have a single "drug problem." We have a heroin problem. We have a problem with marijuana. And with alcohol. And with LSD. And so on. If we are going to solve *any* of these problems, we will have to alter our strategies. Solutions will require that we abandon the slogans and clichés. It will be necessary to do something novel. It will be necessary to *think* about the problems posed by these substances. We will have to ask hard questions up front. We will have to replace glibness with substantive knowledge.

In particular, if we are to find solutions to the problems that cocaine has created, it will be necessary to abandon some long-standing habits of thought. It will be necessary to look for specific information about this specific drug. Programs that work, rather than programs that sound good (and perhaps cost a lot of money), will depend on learning all that it is possible to learn about cocaine: Where does it come from? How is it manufactured? How is it distributed? What does it look like? How do people use it? What are the risk factors in cocaine abuse? Are some people more at risk than others? Where should treatment dollars be spent? On cures? On early intervention? And most important of all, what is it specifically that cocaine does to people who take it?

This is not as easy as it sounds. Easy generalizations must be avoided. Finding out what cocaine does to users is a complicated business. The answer is not in simple catchphrases like "Cocaine really screws you up" or "Cocaine really puts you on top of the world." We need better and more basic information than this. What is needed is detailed information about what cocaine does to people, to their bodies and in particular to their brains. Instead of settling for "Cocaine really screws you up," ask "What is it that cocaine does to the brain that breaks down judgement?" Or, "How does it impair one's ability to consider the consequences of one's actions?" Instead of being content with "Cocaine really puts you on top of the world," ask "What is it that cocaine does to the brain that makes it so difficult to stay away from?"

This information is essential to an understanding of why people take cocaine. Only this type of information will lead us to an understanding of the Helens of this world and of why they are unable to escape the downward spiral of cocaine addiction.

This is an urgent issue. It is purely a matter of luck that our current approach to drugs has not been even *more* of a disaster than it has been. Why luck? Because it was not until recently that cocaine became so readily available to large numbers of our citizens, and because cocaine is *different*. It is different in several important ways from all of the other addictive drugs that have bedeviled our society. Much of this book is concerned with these distinctions. Failure to recognize the unique aspects of cocaine and failure to incorporate this knowledge into our approach to drugs of abuse will guarantee a continued record of failed public policy in the future.

As I will make clear in the next chapter, cocaine is not a new drug on the American scene. It troubled many citizens during earlier periods of our history. It is only in recent years, however, that several factors have combined to turn it into such a potent force in our society. Among these factors are the enormous profits possible from the sale of the drug, the consequent widespread availability, the general loosening, since the sixties, of social constraints on behavior, and the powerful influence of television in transmitting and creating mass culture.

But the bottom line is that these influences have made *cocaine* the force to be reckoned with, and not some other drug. This is not an accident. All of the other drugs of abuse were in place and in a position to assume the role of major player in the drug drama being enacted on our streets. The other drugs are still there. We still have a heroin problem. Marijuana use continues unabated. Amphetamine labs still turn out eagerly awaited supplies of speed. But it is cocaine that has turned this society on its head. It is cocaine that has taxed our law enforcement agencies to the limit and beyond. More than any other force it is cocaine and the billions of dollars that it produces that provide the motives behind money laundering schemes and attempts at payoffs that, if not checked, can threaten the integrity of bedrock institutions like the banks, the judicial system and the police.

Cocaine is different from other drugs. The cocaine epidemic that we are now experiencing is the direct and inevitable result of our failure to acknowledge this difference. We have not acknowledged this difference because we have hidden behind slogans and glib phrases.

A Frightening Look at the Future

Scientific evidence now points to the conclusion that all drugs that produce strong addiction do so because of a similar effect that they produce in the brain. Narcotic drugs, like heroin and morphine, and stimulant drugs, such as amphetamine and cocaine, all seem to affect the brain in related ways. Nevertheless, there are still important differences among them. The similarities and differences are summarized here.

1. Strongly addicting drugs like heroin and cocaine are capable of causing intense feelings of pleasure.
2. These feelings of pleasure result from the ability of the drugs to increase activity in specific parts of the brain.
3. Stimulant drugs like cocaine and amphetamine appear to stimulate these brain areas more directly than do narcotics like heroin and morphine.
4. In both cases, the parts of the brain affected by the drugs are phylogenetically old. That is, they made their appearance early in the process of evolution. Many animal species have similar brain areas.
5. These brain areas have been preserved over millions of years of evolution because they are important ingredients in the ability of individuals and species to adapt and to survive.
6. These areas of the brain are called *pleasure centers* or *reward centers*.

7. The more direct activation by cocaine of these pleasure centers is an important factor in leading people to abuse the drug.
8. Scientists now know a lot about why cocaine is able to do this better than the other drugs. They will know even more about it soon.

This last point provides another important reason for taking a detailed look at cocaine: the development of new drugs. It is very likely that future drugs will include some that are even more destructive than cocaine, more addictive and possibly even more widely available. If we do not begin immediately to approach drugs on an intelligent, rational basis, we will be even less prepared to deal with the new drugs than we have been with cocaine.

In this sense, cocaine provides us with an opportunity. Or, more accurately, it provides us with an imperative. Cocaine confronts us with the fact that drugs are not all alike. Even among drugs of considerable addiction potential, cocaine stands apart. It is, in its various forms, the most destructive drug of abuse in human history. Not heroin, not LSD, not marijuana, not alcohol, not PCP—none of these drugs is as capable as cocaine is of grabbing on and not letting go. If we fail to appreciate this difference, if we do not try to see why it exists, we may be abandoning any realistic hope of coping with new drugs in our future.

The reason that cocaine can exert this powerful hold on people is the unique relationship of the drug to the pleasure centers of the human brain. Cocaine acts, in effect, as a "key" that opens up these parts of the brain as no other drug can do. The nature of this key and the brain functions that it unlocks are examined in detail in the following chapters.

It is of the utmost importance to understand this relationship. Scientists understand it. Pharmacologists understand it. They understand how the key works. And, because they do, they are in a position to make even "better" keys in the future. These keys can and will be made in the laboratory, using all of the sophistication of modern biochemistry and computers. They will be keys to the brain that go beyond cocaine—a better high, a bigger rush. Their products, these keys, will ultimately appear on the street, as have all other drugs of abuse. These products are likely to make current problems with cocaine look simple by comparison. To lump all of these new creations in the category of "drugs," and then to bemoan the fact that our drug problems remain with us, would be a tragic retreat in the face of this challenge.

It would be better to begin now, with cocaine, to ask the hard questions, the penetrating questions. These are questions about the relationship between drugs of abuse and the workings of the brain. It would be better to recognize that the potential exists for making an unlimited number of better cocaine-like keys in the future. Specifically, it is likely that such drugs will be produced at a rate that far outstrips the ability of the legal system to keep up with them. It would be better, in other words, for society, and not just scientists, to appreciate these relationships between drugs and the brain.

The time has come to move beyond slogans. The alternative is a society further benumbed by drugs. The time has come to ask the questions. There is no better place to begin than with cocaine.

A Journey to Understanding

Helen's self-destructive journey into the world of cocaine addiction is not unusual. Cocaine use has reached epidemic proportions in the United States. It is no longer the expensive drug of the wealthy, the favorite "in" drug of Hollywood personalities and professional athletes. The drug, in its various forms, has become quite inexpensive, and its use has permeated all levels of society. It is routinely sold on the streets of our larger cities by thirteen- and fourteen-year-old children. Even nine-year-olds have found that they can make several hundred dollars a week by selling cocaine.

It bears repeating: Helen's story is not unusual. In many ways she is just like the rest of us. She is not a street person of low motivation and meager skills who can find nothing better to do with her time than to pursue her next cocaine high. Neither is she someone with too much money for her own good. Helen is neither a wealthy entertainer nor a star athlete. She was not born with a silver spoon in her mouth.

The fact is that Helen is a striver. A college graduate, near the top of her class, an up-and-coming young professional woman at the beginning of a promising career, she embodies all of the virtues traditionally preached to children in our society. Hard work, determination and self-reliance are integral parts of her character.

Somewhere along the way she stumbled. If you are a cocaine user, you may stumble, too. If you are a "casual" user of the drug, as was Helen when she first started, there is a good chance that you will follow her route and duplicate her experience. That is, no matter how confident you now are of your ability to control your use of cocaine, there is a risk that you will lose control of your drug intake and find your life dominated by cocaine. There is also the very real possibility that you may be even more unlucky than Helen. She survived. You may not.

But, then, why? Why do so many people currently use cocaine? How does cocaine make the user feel? What is it about the drug and the user's reaction to it that makes experiences like Helen's so likely?

In the pages that follow, I will attempt to answer these and many other related questions. Our search for answers will lead us into an exploration of some familiar and much unfamiliar territory. It will entail looking backward five hundred years to the historical events that brought the drug to the attention of Europeans during the Age of Exploration. From this vantage point it will be possible to catch glimpses of events much farther removed in time, legendary events portraying the giving of cocaine to humankind as a gift from beneficent gods. A walk through the troubled streets of the modern city will throw into stark relief the chasm that separates such an exalted conception of the drug's origin from the squalor of the crack house or cocaine shooting gallery.

In order to bridge that chasm, we will follow brief detours that lead through the landscape of the human body. An understanding of how the body is constructed will cast light on how it comes to crave more and more of a simple plant-derived substance. This detour will eventually lead into the recently charted, hidden interior of the human brain. The key to understanding the hold that cocaine is able to exert on the unwary lies here, deep within the brain. Cocaine is able to exert this force because the drug itself is a chemical key that provides entry into basic structures and processes of the brain, processes that are so fundamental to life that they have been conserved over millions of years of evolution.

Chapter 2

A Brief History of a Most Unusual Drug

The year is 1531. For weeks Spanish soldiers under Francisco Pizarro have been climbing ever higher in the Andes Mountains of Peru on a mission of exploration and conquest. Their mission is twofold: bring back the fabled riches of the New World to enrich the coffers of the King of Spain, and provide military support for the missionary priests who will bring back souls for the Holy Catholic Church. The immediate object of their maneuvers is to locate any of the fabulous cities that are reputed to be found at these altitudes.

Pizarro is no newcomer to the New World. Twenty-one years ago he was with Vasco Nuñez de Balboa when European adventurers first set eyes on the Pacific Ocean. Based in Panama since then, he has carried out extensive explorations of the country to the south of the isthmus. He has organized and participated in two long and difficult sea voyages down the west coast of South America. In the course of these explorations, Pizarro has learned of a new civilization centered in Peru. His brief but tantalizing glimpses of this civilization during his coastal explorations, and the incredible stories told to him by the natives, have convinced him that this new kingdom, this kingdom of the Incas, will rival the Aztec Empire in importance and wealth. He is convinced that his fame, and particularly his fortune, will be guaranteed if he can return and conquer this Indian civilization in the name of the Spanish king.

And so, in 1528, he returns to Spain to plead his case. He is eloquent and persuasive. King Charles I of Spain, the Holy Roman Emperor Charles V, grants Pizarro's request that he be allowed to conquer and rule the ancient civilization of the Incas. And why should the king not be pleased with such a plan? Since the initial discoveries of Columbus, Spain has done exceedingly well in this business of building empires. Cortez has subjugated Mexico, taking the first steps to insure that the wealth of that country will flow to Spain. Why not extend the empire ever farther to the south? Why not conquer another empire that may even surpass the Aztec Empire in gold and riches? Bold men, fearless men like Pizarro, are available and, with minimal financing, seem to be able to make short work of it.

Pizarro and the soldiers in his army are not interested in the larger questions of building empires. They are preoccupied with gold, silver and jewels—the rewards of conquest that will bring them honor and wealth. This is why the hardships are endured. The prospect of finding such riches has supplanted the original impetus for exploration of the New World—the search for a shorter route to the Orient and the treasures found there.

Seen from our present vantage point, there is an element of irony in all of this. In the green foliage surrounding these soldiers is a source of riches far greater than the gold they seek. This plant-derived source of wealth is of greater potential value than the highly sought-after spice plants, the search for which initiated the exploration of this new world. The extent of this wealth is beyond the comprehension of the individual soldier. He would scoff at the suggestion that these plants and their products would one day be fought over by private armies waging private wars on several continents. He would find it incredible that the commanders of these armies would control financial resources sufficient to corrupt sovereign nations. And he would find it beyond belief that the most powerful nation on earth, thousands of miles distant from this site, would one day consider dedicating a significant portion of its armed might to establishing control over the production and distribution of these plants.

The plants are the source of cocaine, the plant now called the coca plant. The biologist Jean-Baptiste de Lamarck would, two hundred years later, make this classification official when he designated the plant *Erythroxylon coca*. The plant should be not confused with the cocao plant, from which chocolate is obtained, nor with the coconut plant, a species of palm tree. It is only the coca plant that yields cocaine, and this has made it a source of great wealth. This potential wealth has caused the bitter present-day struggle to control the cultivation of the plant and the distribution of the product that it yields. Governments bicker and feud over these questions. Vast criminal empires wage war over several continents in an effort to establish dominance of the cocaine trade. The coca plant, which was introduced to the Europeans through the bloody ravages of the conquistadores, lies today at the root of the bloody battles being waged on the streets of American cities.

The history of cocaine from the sixteenth century until the present day is filled with heroism and treachery, conquest and subjugation, scientific triumph and failure, medical hope and despair. Perhaps most of all it is a history of human frailty. While the entire story of cocaine is too long to be told here, it cannot be ignored altogether. The major events that are essential to an understanding of the problem of cocaine in America today need to be told.

Before Pizarro, in the fifteenth century, several European explorers had returned telling of the use of coca leaves by the inhabitants of the New World. It is with the Spanish conquest of the Inca civilization in South American in the sixteenth century, however, that the European infatuation with cocaine begins. The local Indians set great store by this plant and told marvelous stories of its origins. Some of these stories linked the plant to sexual prowess and fertility. Other legends revealed that the plant was evidence of a special relationship between these people and their god. The legends claimed it had initially been a gift to them from a benevolent god who viewed them with special favor. The plant was associated with rituals and ceremonies that testified to this special character.

According to some of the accounts, the use of the coca plant in preconquest times had been restricted much more than when the conquistadores arrived on the scene. It seems that earlier in history the plant could be used only by the emperor and his royal family. The emperor was a godlike figure to his people, and he enjoyed a privileged relationship to the coca plant that was in keeping with this divine connection. He could exert strict control over its use by his subjects. So strict was his control, and so sought after was the coca plant, that the emperor was able to use its distribution as a form of social control. From time to time he could distribute some of it to his subjects as a reward for particularly valuable service.

By the time of the Spanish conquest, however, restrictions on the use of the plant had been considerably relaxed, and its use was more widespread. Even though the connection with the emperor and the gods had been weakened, the plant continued to enjoy a favored status. Naturally, the Spaniards were curious. These early sixteenth-century Europeans lived in an age when faith was beginning to yield to science in explaining natural phenomena. Little was known about the origin of disease, and even less about its cure, and belief in the supernatural, in miracles, was still widespread. They were quite naturally interested in stories of a wondrous plant of possible divine origin. What was this plant, they wondered, and what was it used for?

The Indians used the coca plant in several different situations. They used it as a stimulant, chewing the leaves to banish fatigue. In the harsh environment of higher altitudes, this stimulant enabled the Indians to work harder and longer without complaining, and without tiring. The plant was also used to measure time and distance. It was common practice for the Indians to describe a journey in terms of the number of mouthfuls of leaves that normally would be chewed in making the trip.

The conquerors quickly saw the advantage of controlling its distribution. They, too, used the coca plant as a reward. The Spaniards now played the role of emperor, using the coca plant as an incentive to increase the output of forced native labor. Control of its distribution became one of the weapons wielded by the conquistadores in their conquest of the Inca empire.

Of more immediate interest, however, is the fact that the Spanish brought these tales home with them. Their accounts from this period aroused curiosity in Europe. In 1596, a Spanish physician, Nicolas Monardes, published the first paper on the effects of the coca plant. For the next two hundred years, European interest in the plant surfaced periodically. Most of this interest was botanical in focus, culminating with its "official" classification by Lamarck in 1783.

From Plant to Drug: The Emergence of a Scourge

About another hundred years would elapse following Lamarck's work before the coca plant would generate more interest on the European scene. The resurgence came first through medicine. Physicians wondered if this exotic plant could be used to treat disease. Many other plants had found their way into medicine. Perhaps this new plant would provide new treatments, even cures, for the ailments and afflictions of the time. Popular interest in the plant soon followed, for popular interest and medical treatment blended easily in the public mind. By the middle of the nineteenth century this combination of medical and popular interest in the coca plant had resulted in its inclusion as an ingredient in numerous tonics and medications. The best known of these preparations was a wine, Vin Mariani, produced in Europe by Angelo Mariani. Its use soon spread to the United States. Numerous physicians testified to its efficacy in treating various kinds of illness. Other coca-based patent medicines appeared and were promoted for use in treating a range of maladies, including venereal disease, dysentery, narcotic addiction and alcoholism.

Experimentation with the plant in these preparations led naturally to the question of what was in the plant that enabled it to act as it did. It was only a matter of time until cocaine was isolated and identified as the active ingredient in the plant. This isolation of the active agent began the transformation of the ancient herb of the Incas into the drug that is so intertwined with our contemporary social and political fabric. While there is some dispute over who should be given credit for the isolation of cocaine (some say that the honor should go to Friedrich Gaedecke while others say it should go to Albert Niemann), the fact is that by 1860 cocaine was known to be the active ingredient that caused the effects the plant produced. As a result, medical investigators had a ready source of pure chemical to experiment with. They now possessed control over the dose they administered, a degree of certainty they did not have in their previous investigations using crude extracts of plant leaves.

And investigate they did! Cocaine soon came to be regarded in many quarters as a "wonder drug" that was potentially able to cure many illnesses. The drug was pressed into service on many fronts in the ongoing battle against the host of real and imagined ills that beset mankind. In the short time between the isolation of pure cocaine from the coca plant and the beginning of awareness of its undesirable side effects, cocaine was used almost everywhere. There were few conditions that did not receive at least passing consideration as candidates for treatment with cocaine. As the results of these initial investigations appeared in print, medical authorities and the public alike uncritically embraced the new drug and the extravagant claims of its benefits.

One of the first attempts to use the newly available drug was made in a military setting. The German physician Theodor Aschenbrandt in 1883 administered cocaine to soldiers on maneuvers with the Bavarian army. Could he use the drug, he wondered, to increase their endurance under battle conditions? His experiment harked back to the earliest reports of the stimulant characteristics of the coca plant. He probably was also familiar with the reports of the military use of the coca plant for stimulant purposes among the defenders of La Paz a century earlier. Aschenbrandt's report, in a German medical journal, of the stimulant effect of the drug on his soldiers is one of the first reports to bring cocaine to the attention of a wider medical audience.

From the Battlefield to the Clinic

The major significance of Aschenbrandt's experiment, however, lies not in its military applications, but rather in the fact that his report was read by a young Viennese neurologist. The neurologist was intrigued enough by Aschenbrandt's report to secure some of the drug for himself and to begin experimentation with it. His reports were to be instrumental in bringing cocaine to the notice of a larger audience and in heightening public curiosity about the drug.

The neurologist was Sigmund Freud, who would later achieve fame as the founder of psychoanalysis. At this time, however, he had not yet begun his psychoanalytic work. He was, instead, a rather unsuccessful medical practitioner, not well off financially, and apparently determined to discover or create something that would bring him fame and fortune. His reading of the Aschenbrandt report meshed with his reading of several other reports from American sources concerning possible medical applications of cocaine. While Freud is remembered by most people for his psychological theorizing and his invention of psychoanalysis, his publications from this period on cocaine mark him as a major player in the history of this drug.

One of his interests lay in the problems that his friend and fellow physician Ernst von Fleischl was having with morphine. Fleischl had become addicted to morphine after using it to treat himself for a chronically painful condition involving tumors of the peripheral nerves. Freud thought he could use cocaine to break Fleischl's addiction to morphine. He gave the drug to Fleischl and was pleased to note that, indeed, cocaine became more important to him than morphine had been. Much to Freud's chagrin and alarm, however, Fleischl was soon to exceed Freud's prescribed amount of the drug, and before long he was injecting it in amounts of up to a gram a day. Fleischl progressed from insomnia and restlessness to hallucinations and convulsions. Many of his nights were spent in terror of imaginary white snakes crawling over his skin. Rather than a medical triumph, Freud had given birth to the first well-documented case of cocaine psychosis.

Freud had also tried the drug himself, at a time when he was undergoing a low period in his life. Cocaine lifted his spirits and took his mind off his personal and professional difficulties. Listen to the words of the man who was destined to be the most influential psychiatrist of the first half of the twentieth century: "I take very small doses of it regularly against depression and against indigestion, and with the most brilliant success." And in sending cocaine to his fiancée, he told her it would "make [her] strong and give [her] cheeks a red color."

As a result of his personal experiences, Freud became, for a time, an unabashed promoter of the drug. He wrote several articles for medical journals suggesting that cocaine might be used in treating a variety of ills, including asthma, digestive upset and morphine addiction, among others. He even suggested that cocaine might be used as an aphrodisiac. He encouraged his fellow physicians to try the drug. He told his sister and his fiancée that the drug had made him a new man and he encouraged them to try it themselves. When, toward the end of the nineteenth century, medical opinion was awakening to the dangers and limitations of the drug, Freud continued his defense of cocaine. For example, it was not until pressures against his advocacy greatly increased that, in 1887, Freud abandoned his suggestion that cocaine could be used to treat morphine addiction. Even then he suggested that the failures were not cocaine's. Failures were the result, he said, of the weak will which he claimed was characteristic of the morphine abuser.

(In the early years of the twentieth century, medical opinion became increasingly critical of cocaine. Publications in medical journals in this country and in Europe in the years prior to World War I had discredited most uses of the drug, a major exception being its use as a local anesthetic.)

In Freud's chapter in the history of cocaine are found most of the themes that will be repeated time and again as society learns and relearns the facts of cocaine use. The euphoriant effects of the drug that are the immediate objective of the cocaine user are described by Freud in his personal use of the drug. The development of compulsive use of the drug is evident in the spectacle of Fleischl's inability to control his intake. And the insistence by Freud, in the face of accumulating evidence to the contrary, that cocaine is a beneficial drug that has virtually no downside to it is a litany that can be heard over and over today by apologists for cocaine.

The American Connection

In the history of cocaine, Freud is an important figure for yet another reason. He participated in the events leading up to the discovery of the one valid medical use of cocaine, namely, its use as a local anesthetic. Freud, like others before him, noticed a tingling of the lips and tongue when cocaine was applied there. He used the words "anesthetic property," referring to cocaine, in an essay written in 1884. In an autobiography written years later, Freud suggests that he might have gone on to investigate this further if other events had not distracted him. He acknowledges that his friend and fellow physician, Carl Koller, did the necessary experiments to demonstrate cocaine's effect as a local anesthetic. While he proposes that Koller should be regarded as the discoverer of this property of the drug, Freud points out that he himself had suggested this direction of research to Koller.

Through an interest in the local anesthetic properties of cocaine another major player enters the stage, one of the giants of American medicine, William Halstead. Halstead is often called the Father of

American Surgery. One of the four distinguished founders of The Johns Hopkins Medical School, his experiments with cocaine led to an intense addiction that threatened his illustrious career. The addiction developed when he was a young physician making a name for himself in New York City in the latter half of the nineteenth century. When he started his experiments, cocaine was recognized as a good surface anesthetic (as in the cornea of the eye). Halstead wanted to see how far he could take the idea of cocaine-induced anesthesia. He injected the drug in the vicinity of a nerve to see if a deeper, but still local, anesthesia could be produced. Such an anesthesia would be limited to those nerves affected directly by the cocaine. If this local anesthesia went deep enough, surgery could be performed. The advantages of such surgery are many, including the fact that the patient does not have to be rendered unconscious with a general anesthetic. Halstead was successful in this regard, and the methods that he developed, beginning in the late 1880s, mark the beginning of surgical procedures using local rather than general anesthetics.

Unfortunately, his success was not without cost to himself and to several of his colleagues. It was not uncommon at the time for scientists to use themselves as guinea pigs in their research. Halstead injected himself frequently with cocaine in the preliminary stages of his investigations, and this is where Halstead the Scientist got derailed by Halstead the Man. While Halstead the Scientist may have been interested in the anesthetic properties of cocaine, Halstead the Man could only respond to the enticing nature of the drug. As his intellect was evaluating the local anesthetic action of the drug, the rest of his body was telling him only how good cocaine made him feel. The result was that he developed a craving for the drug that he could not master.

Halstead tried desperately to overcome his desire for cocaine. He knew that his career was threatened. Aware that he could not give up the drug when it was readily available, he attempted to isolate himself from it. He tried secluding himself for an extended period in a mountain cabin where he would not have access to the drug. His friends took him on a long cruise to the Caribbean to help him wean himself from cocaine. He was hospitalized on two separate occasions. None of these efforts succeeded in breaking the cocaine habit until, finally, after the second hospitalization, he was able to give up his use of cocaine. At last, free of his dependence on cocaine, he went on to pursue one of the distinguished careers in American medicine.

Halstead's saga may at first glance seem to be testimony to the triumph of the human will over the grip of an addicting drug. His story might be taken to demonstrate that determination is sufficient to break the grip of cocaine addiction. Reality suggests otherwise, however. For in later years it would be revealed that Halstead, to battle the uncontrollable craving for cocaine, had turned to morphine. Morphine helped to subdue the insistent urge to inject himself with cocaine. Halstead switched his addiction from cocaine to morphine. And the "treatment" was not temporary or short-term. He seems to have remained addicted to morphine throughout much or all of the remainder of his productive life.

It is worth noting that such negative consequences of cocaine use in medical settings gave rise to an interest in finding substitute drugs. In particular, a search was launched to find local anesthetics that would not have the extreme addiction potential of cocaine. The search was successful, of course, and the use of drugs such as Novocaine in dentistry is well known. Cocaine is still used in very restricted medical circumstances, such as in some cases of ophthalmological surgery. With few exceptions, however, it has been replaced by drugs without cocaine's addictive properties.

Some People Never Get the Word

The story of cocaine during the late nineteenth and early twentieth centuries is, unfortunately, not simply a tale of scientists and medical practitioners. It was an age in which patent medicines and over-the-counter nostrums proliferated, much as they do today. Legislation regulating the production and sale of such preparations, however, was still several years away. Over-the-counter preparations containing morphine, codeine, opium and cocaine were widely available, and they required no prescription. They were used by many people.

Cocaine appeared in preparations sold as "tonics," in which ground coca leaves constituted the most important ingredient. These products sold well and were frequently promoted and ballyhooed with the endorsements of famous personalities of the era. Coca-Cola took half of its name from one of the most important ingredients in its initial formulation. The cocaine was removed from the prototypical American soft drink, however, shortly before the passage in 1907 of the Pure Food and Drug Act. (It is interesting to note that this legislation would not have required the removal of cocaine from the drink, but would have required that its presence be listed on the label. In this sense, the legislation was not a prohibitive act.)

Pure cocaine, the drug itself—not mixed in tonics or other preparations—was quick to appear in nonmedical circles. Almost immediately after the isolation of cocaine, the drug made its appearance in the larger culture, and with devastating effect. The agony that Helen experienced with the drug, and the moments of ecstasy she was seeking when she started using it, have been experienced by many before her. Indeed, among the people who anticipated her experience are some quite illustrious names from the fields of science, the arts and letters. It will be informative to review a bit of their testimony.

Sir Arthur Conan Doyle's "Sign of Four" was written only two years after the isolation of pure cocaine from the coca plant. The accuracy of the portrayal of Sherlock Holmes's use of cocaine suggests that the drug had already become well known.

> Sherlock Holmes took his bottle from the corner of the mantelpiece, and his hypodermic syringe from its neat morocco case. With his long, white nervous fingers, he adjusted the delicate needle and rolled back his left shirtcuff. For some little time his eyes rested thoughtfully upon the sinewy forearm and wrist, all dotted and scarred with innumerable puncture-marks. Finally, he thrust the sharp point home, pressed down the tiny piston, and sank back into the velvet-lined armchair with a long sigh of satisfaction.
>
> Three times a day for many months I had witnessed this performance, but custom had not reconciled my mind to it. On the contrary, from day to day I had become more irritable at the sight, and my conscience swelled nightly within me at the thought that I had lacked the courage to protest . . .
>
> "Which is it today," I asked, "Morphine or cocaine?"
>
> He raised his eyes languidly from the old black-letter volume which he had opened.
>
> "It is cocaine," he said, "a seven-per-cent solution. Would you care to try it?"

"No, indeed," I answered brusquely. "My constitution has not got over the Afghan campaign yet. I cannot afford to throw any extra strain upon it."

He smiled at my vehemence. "Perhaps you are right, Watson," he said. "I suppose that its influence is physically a bad one. I find it, however, so transcendently stimulating and clarifying to the mind that its secondary action is a matter of small moment."

"But consider!" I said earnestly. "Count the cost! Your brain may, as you say, be roused and excited, but it is a pathological and morbid process which involves increased tissue-change and may at least leave a permanent weakness. You know, too, what a black reaction comes upon you. Surely the game is hardly worth the candle. Why should you, for a mere passing pleasure, risk the loss of those great powers with which you have been endowed? Remember that I speak not only as one comrade to another but as a medical man . . ."

He did not seem offended. On the contrary, he put his finger-tips together, and leaned his elbows on the arms of his chair, like one who has a relish for conversation.

"My mind," he said, "rebels at stagnation. Give me problems, give me work, give me the most abstruse cryptogram, or the most intricate analysis, and I am in my own proper atmosphere. I can dispense then with artificial stimulants. But I abhor the dull routine of existence. I crave for mental exaltation . . ."

In a similar vein, an article in an American medical journal in the early 1970s examined the possibility that Robert Louis Stevenson may have written "Dr. Jekyll and Mr. Hyde" while under the influence of cocaine. While there is no certain documentation of this, several interesting facts are known. Stevenson was at the time ill with tuberculosis, an illness for which he had been taking morphine. It is likely that cocaine also would have been prescribed for him. During the period when Stevenson was writing, cocaine was used widely in attempts to cure or alleviate a broad range of illness. While it is not certain that he used cocaine, it is well known that he was able to sustain an intense level of activity while writing the book. He wrote two drafts of the novel, a production of about 60,000 words, in a period of only six days!

In the late nineteenth and early twentieth centuries cocaine figured prominently in the larger culture. The undiluted, pure drug was widely known and used. Witness the reference to it in Cole Porter's "I Get a Kick Out of You," a popular song of the day:

> I get no kick from cocaine
> I'm sure that if
> I took even one sniff
> It would bore me terrifically, too
> But I get a kick out of you.

Other individuals from the past can be called upon to testify to the widespread knowledge of cocaine in times before our own. Some of them, like Helen, reached a crisis stage where their use of cocaine had spiraled out of control. Others had faced the necessity of trying to guide their friends through the perils of cocaine addiction. In all cases, the users sought, initially, the exhilaration of a cocaine "high," the pleasurable intensity of which has been described as better than sexual orgasm. They shared also the initial conviction that the drug was "safe," the conviction that they could control its use and not experience any undesired consequences. The fact that so many people could be so badly misled is testimony to the strength of the drive for pleasure in the human species, as well as to the remarkable human tendency to resist letting the cautionary advice of others interfere with this quest.

But why should the larger culture *not* look to cocaine to cure its ills? After all, the Parke-Davis Pharmaceutical Company noted in 1885 that the drug could "supply the place of food, make the coward brave, and the silent eloquent . . ."

While cocaine during the early twentieth century was never used to the extent it would be in the 1980s, its use was nonetheless quite widespread. Between 1887 and 1914 forty-six states passed some form of legislation aimed at controlling it. This legislative activity is testimony to a popular awareness that the drug posed a significant problem for society.

Several factors combined finally to reduce the extent of cocaine use in the United States. In 1914, the federal government mistakenly classified cocaine as a narcotic, which it is not, and outlawed its use with the passage of the Harrison Narcotic Act. This legislation made cocaine available only by physician's prescription. Probably an even greater contributor to the decline of cocaine use during this period was cocaine's increasingly bad press. The drug was frequently associated in the general public's mind with the lower social classes, blacks and criminals, but its use among society's elite went unremarked or ignored. Cries for its control were at least in a part a cry for control of what were seen by many people to be the less desirable segments of society.

Law enforcement's attempts to root out drug use increased during the prohibition era of the 1920s, and cocaine use declined. The decline was aided and abetted during the 1930s by an unexpected development. Amphetamine use became increasingly common among drug users during this period and significantly eroded the popularity of cocaine. Amphetamine had several characteristics that were appealing to the cocaine aficionado. It produced a "high" very much like cocaine's. It did not deliver quite the same peak intensity, but its effects lasted longer. More significantly, the new drug was cheap and readily available. With the appearance of large amounts of legally obtainable amphetamine, cocaine use declined appreciably. Its use remained low until a shift in law enforcement priorities in the 1960s made amphetamine more difficult to obtain. Drug dealers and users switched back to the neglected cocaine and the first flurries of the current blizzard arrived.

From this brief history it is possible to draw several conclusions that will help in understanding the role that cocaine plays in our society today. First, cocaine is not a drug that burst anew upon the scene sometime in the 1960s. It has been known in medical circles and in the popular culture for more than a century. Second, the major dangers of cocaine were known almost from the very first uses of the purified drug. Its use in medicine, once the naive enthusiasm for the "wonder drug" had been tempered by experience, has been largely restricted to producing local anesthesia. And even in this area, the dangers of cocaine led to the early substitution of safer drugs.

The major undesirable side effects of the medical use of cocaine are the euphoria it produces and the overwhelming tendency it has to create strong dependence and addiction. Drugs that "turn people on" or produce euphoria as a side effect are regarded with caution by the medical community. The reason is obvious. Such drugs are liable to be taken by patients in increasing amounts for reasons quite incidental to the medical reasons for their use. Such drugs are, in other words, likely to be abused and are likely to be addicting. The classic example is found in the opiates, like morphine. As pain relievers they are without peer, and modern medicine would be unthinkable without them. They are used with caution, however, because they can lead to addiction. It is essential to note that, in the case of cocaine, the "undesirable" medical side effects of euphoria and exhilaration are exactly the effects deliberately sought by the casual user and the addicted individual.

Chapter 3

The Different Faces of Paradise

In spite of the lessons of the past, cocaine today constitutes the most troubling of our drug problems. The recreational use of cocaine is higher today than at any other time in our history. The number of casualties ascribed to its use is rising, with no certainty that the peak is in sight. The incidence of cocaine-related violent crime has reached unbelievably high levels. The amount of illicit money pouring into the coffers of criminal organizations is beyond the comprehension of most of us. Experts believe that organized crime receives more than half its income from illegal drug dealings, to the tune of $10 to $50 *billion* per year. We know that illicit drug profits have been instrumental in the corruption of officials in Latin America. This vast store of money has been said to be responsible for increasing amounts of corruption at various levels of our own criminal justice system.

Our cocaine problem has led to foreign policy initiatives that would see us clamoring for war if such actions were directed against us by a foreign power. We have tried to redefine our own problem of unrelenting consumption into a problem of foreign production. We have attempted to dictate to other sovereign nations, typically small and powerless, what cash crops they may produce. In the name of cocaine control we have attempted to destroy, or have destroyed, the coca plants that are the main source of income of many of the small farmers and peasants in these countries. We have connived in the illegal kidnapping on foreign soil of foreign nationals whom we suspect of trafficking in cocaine. Imagine the call to action that would be heard in this country if we were similarly treated by a foreign power. Imagine the call to action if other nations threatened us with reprisals unless we stopped growing and exporting tobacco. It is a virtual certainty that we would regard all such protestations as unacceptable meddling in our internal affairs.

And yet all of these foreign policy entanglements may not be the most significant aspect of the destruction wrought by cocaine. The most enduring legacy of cocaine may prove to be, if we are not careful, an undermining of our nation's basic democratic institutions. The futility of our attempts to suppress the demand for and the distribution of cocaine has pushed us dangerously close to abandoning long-standing, cherished civil liberties in a last-ditch attempt to assert control. In the name of cocaine control, we are perilously close to empowering the military with the right to stop, search and seize civilians on the streets of our country. In the name of cocaine control, we, as a society, are on the brink of handing over to the military a degree of control over American civilians that until now we thought existed only in military dictatorships. All of this in a country dedicated to individual liberty and the supremacy of civil authority over the military.

Why?

Why should one drug, a very simple chemical, be able to exert such a profound and pervasive influence on our people and our institutions? Where have we gone wrong? All of our attempts to cope with this particular drug problem have been dismal failures. The politicians who make our drug policies and the bureaucrats in charge of implementing those policies, however, do not know that or will not admit it. Our problems with cocaine have intensified in direct proportion to the amount of money we have spent in trying to solve these problems.

We have tried valiantly to reduce the amount of cocaine coming into the country. Hardly a night goes by without a television report of another big drug bust. We've read the headlines so often that they no longer make an impression. "Federal agents seize massive cocaine shipment. Street value placed at 100 million dollars." A few years ago, when we first read such reports, we could feel encouraged. Vigilant law enforcement seemed to be removing significant quantities of a dangerous drug from our streets. More recently, however, we've come to realize that all of these praiseworthy efforts have scarcely made a dent in the supply of cocaine on our streets. No matter how many cocaine shipments are seized, no matter how many tons of cocaine are turned back at our borders, no matter how many drug rings are broken up, the supply does not dry up. The drug doesn't go away.

On the demand side our failures have been almost equally depressing. "Let's just educate people on the problems and dangers associated with cocaine use. Let's dry up the demand for the drug." More recently, "Education won't do the job. We have to punish the drug user as well as the drug seller. That's it! Get tough, real tough! How about zero tolerance? Let's put an end to this drug craving once and for all." And with what result? While we may have made some small progress in reducing demand through education, there is still plenty of demand to go around. The drug runners are, after all, not making their profits selling the drug to one another. They have customers. While we may have succeeded in teaching a few people to "just say no," millions of others continue to respond with a resounding "yes!"

Why have we failed in our legal approaches to rid our streets of cocaine? Why have our educational efforts not been more successful in reducing the demand for the drug? Why, instead, have we seen the appearance on our streets of new and more destructive forms of cocaine? The answer was suggested in the first chapter: *We don't know the enemy.* As a society we do not understand what we are up against. As a society we have not asked for, and our leaders have not seen fit to give us, enough information about the problem. The simple solutions we have tried have not worked.

The failure of simplistic solutions, in the absence of any real knowledge of the enemy, can lead us into dangers that are far worse than those produced by the drug itself. Consider in a little more detail the questions of how to disrupt supply and reduce demand. These are public policy questions of the utmost importance. These questions are important because the way that we answer them can take us right to the core of our shared ideas of what democracy, individual freedom and the collective good are all about. Indeed, such questions, if seriously pursued, have the potential for illuminating, for better or worse, the extent to which we do or do not have a consensus in this country about these core values.

Consider, for example, the reduction of demand. Almost everyone would agree that this is a good idea. But, how do we go about reducing demand? More effective educational efforts? Certainly. Almost everyone would agree with that. But, then again, almost everyone would agree that more effective educational efforts alone will not completely eliminate the demand. Additional steps are likely to be needed.

From here on, unfortunately, agreement may be a little bit harder to come by. Should we initiate mandatory drug testing for our citizens? Make no mistake about it, mandatory drug testing, and the implied penalties (loss of job, prison term) that would be imposed on anyone testing positive, would definitely put a crimp in the demand for cocaine. However, getting agreement that such testing should be done, and on what scale and to whom, is not so easy. The question is wildly controversial because it places in the balance two highly valued societal objectives and forces us to choose between them. The values weighed are a drug-free society on the one hand, and individual liberty on the other. If we choose mandatory testing, we turn our backs on the cherished right of a free people to be secure. This right of a free people goes by several names: freedom from unwarranted search and seizure, freedom from self-incrimination. We Americans think highly of these freedoms. We fought a war of independence to secure them and other freedoms that we consider to be the birthright of a free people.

If you think that the choice is not quite that difficult, that the alternatives need not be quite that sharply drawn, ask yourself how we would choose who is to be tested. Is everyone to be tested? If so, how often? And by whom? Not very practical, you say. Besides, we all know that testing everyone would require a government apparatus so large and so intrusive that individual liberties would rapidly disappear into its ravening maw.

Well, then, perhaps only those of us who occupy "sensitive" and "critical" positions in our culture should be routinely tested. People like airline pilots, policemen and physicians. Maybe that's a promising approach. But just who is to make the judgment about what is a "sensitive" or a "critical" position? Our lawmakers, our elected representatives, of course. But what about those elected representatives? The congressmen and the senators who make our laws and who frequently have access to important national security information hold positions of high trust. Are these not "sensitive" positions? Do we want to entrust our national security and the framing of our laws to a collection of drug-addled individuals who can't think straight? Shouldn't these individuals, perhaps more than any others, be subject to mandatory testing, perhaps as a precondition for holding office? Why not demand that anyone wishing to run for public office be tested for drugs before he can become a candidate? And if he is elected, should he not be tested routinely thereafter? There is not likely to be much agreement here.

On the other side of the ledger, questions about how to disrupt supply can lead us to answers which shape our view of the world in which we live. In answering them we are fully capable of defining which nations are to be our friends and which nations are to be our enemies. It has happened before in history. Wars have been fought over the distribution of drugs. The Opium War fought by the British against the Chinese is one example. It is not too difficult to imagine a scenario which finds us similarly entangled with a foreign power over the issue of drug distribution. In the attempt to stop cocaine at our borders we could easily move to stop the drug before it gets to our borders. We could destroy the fields in distant countries where the drug is grown. We could stop ships on the high seas, foreign flag carriers as well as our own, and search them for cocaine. These are not peaceful actions taken against foreign nationals and their governments.

Fortunately, there are other roads to follow if we are wise enough to seek them out. They all depend on asking some hard questions at the outset. And these questions must be asked dispassionately, in an open-minded way that does not cut off debate. Above all, an attempt must be made to avoid polemics. One of the reasons we have not done a better job in solving the cocaine problem is that the issues themselves get lost in the discussion. Drug abuse is a topic that can be counted on to generate a debate that forces people into fixed, preconceived positions. And in this arena there *are* rigidly fixed positions. At one extreme are adherents to the view that anything that has been labeled a drug (not a "medicine") is evil. Its users are evil, too, and should be dealt with most severely. At the other extreme are adherents to the view that anything that is called a drug is good. Its users are enlightened beings who should be left alone to pursue their own higher truth. There is little real communication between the holders of these views. "I'll believe the evidence that I bring to the discussion. You can believe yours, if you choose. But, don't try to confuse me. My mind's made up." Much of our drug debate at the public policy level has this character to it. The debate has generated a lot more heat than light.

The novel idea I am introducing here is that we should begin by trying to learn as much as possible about cocaine. The notion is simple. If our object is to arrive at policies and programs that can free society of the devastating effects of cocaine, we really do have to know something about the enemy. We have to begin by learning all we can about the drug itself and about the ways in which the drug produces its effects on the body and on the mind. Only when we have a clear understanding of the effects of the drug, and the way in which it produces these effects, only then will we meet with any success in finding solutions to problems it creates.

There is something else to be gained from this approach. With any luck it will "take." Perhaps we can learn to adopt it as a general strategy. If so, if we can get into the habit of demanding good, solid information about the drugs that bedevil our society, we will be in a much better position to solve the problems that they create. This type of enlightened approach will be indispensable the future, in the years beyond cocaine.

A Rose Is Not a Rose Is Not a Rose . . .

A good way to start the process is at the beginning. Cocaine, as discussed in the last chapter, is derived from the coca plant. It is important to realize that it is not the plant itself that is at the root of our current problems. It is, rather, one constituent of the plant, cocaine, extracted in highly purified form, that causes the difficulty. This is not an idle distinction. This is not merely wordplay; the distinction is important.

For hundreds of years prior to the purification of cocaine, South American Indians chewed the leaves of the coca plant. Chewing the leaves liberated the cocaine contained in them and made it available for use by the body. Early observers of this practice noted that Indians who regularly chewed coca in the higher elevation of the Andes Mountains could, and regularly did, give up the practice when they moved to lower altitudes. Even though they were using cocaine, in other words, they did not show the signs of extreme drug dependence that we see in our time and culture. While the reasons for this lack of dependence may not be entirely clear, the observation suggests, at least, that there may be important differences between the cocaine taken by these Indians as they chewed their leaves and the cocaine used today. Another way to put it is that serious thinking about problems with cocaine might well start with some questions about the *form* of the drug.

The first question then is, "What are the various forms in which cocaine is sold and used?" Here, we must focus on the processes involved in removing the drug from its plant source. Modern chemistry does a much better job of this than does the chewer of coca leaves. Not surprisingly, the real problems with cocaine did not begin until the chemists figured out how to isolate it from its plant base.

Cocaine is what chemists call an alkaloid. Although this term may not be familiar to the layman, everyone is familiar with alkaloids. Caffeine, for example, is an alkaloid of the coffee bean. Nicotine is an alkaloid found in the tobacco plant. Plants that contain alkaloids frequently contain a number of similar but distinct alkaloids. Usually, only one, or at most a few, of these will be of any biological interest. The hemp plant from which marijuana comes, for example, contains numerous alkaloids similar to THC, the alkaloid that causes the characteristic effects of marijuana smoke, but THC is the only one that is of any interest as a drug.

The first job, therefore, in learning how a plant produces its effects is to find a way to remove these alkaloids from the plant, purify them, and test them to see which one produces the effects in question. At this point, alkaloids like cocaine can be purified and separated from other, unwanted components of the plant by chemical means. The basic procedure is an extraction. During this process the plant leaves are soaked in various chemical solvents. The process involves several steps, but the essential result is that the cocaine is drawn out of the leaves and into the solvent. The cocaine can then be removed from the solvent by additional chemical means and obtained in a pure form, free of contaminants.

In the lengthy multistep procedure used in the legal extraction of cocaine from the coca plant, the leaves are first crushed and alcohol is percolated through them to remove the crude, unpurified alkaloids from the leaves. The alcohol at this point also contains additional waxy material from the leaves, which is removed by heating and cooling the alcohol mixture, a process that solidifies the unwanted wax. In the next step the alkaloids are removed from the alcohol by sequential washings with acid and basic mixtures. The removed alkaloids are then treated with kerosene, yielding cocaine which is about 60 percent pure.

There is a problem with the cocaine at this point, however. It does not dissolve well in water. This means that the drug in this form cannot be used for injection into the bloodstream, because human blood is about 50 percent water. Any drug which is injected into the bloodstream must be dissolvable in water—if it is not, it will just float around the body in a nondissolved clump. Such clumps are likely to cause strokes or cardiac arrest. Because of factors like these, the extracted cocaine is further treated with oxidizing agents and acids to produce a water-soluble form of the drug. This form of the drug is about 99 percent pure cocaine.

Figure 3.1 shows these relationships among the various forms of

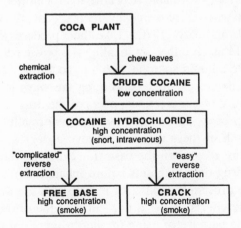

Fig. 3.1 Various forms of cocaine obtained from the coca plant, and typical methods of use

cocaine. Other forms of cocaine (free base and crack) are also shown in this figure.

It may seem that the methods involved in producing cocaine would present insurmountable obstacles to the illegal manufacture of the drug. Nothing could be further from the truth. The illegal manufacturer of cocaine may use somewhat simplified equipment, but the procedures he uses are very similar to those described above. Alcohol percolation to extract the crude alkaloids is followed by acid-base washings to precipitate the crude cocaine. Kerosene baths and chilling are used to isolate the cocaine further. In this fashion, illegal cocaine laboratories are easily able to turn out cocaine that is more than 90 percent pure. The manufacture of the drug from its plant source is among the least of the problems confronting the illegal producer of the drug.

The final form of cocaine normally obtained by these procedures is *cocaine hydrochloride.* Cocaine in this form is referred to by the chemist as a *salt.* It is very stable, and has the appearance of a white, crystalline powder. Until very recently, cocaine hydrochloride was the only type of cocaine known on the streets or in medical practice. And almost from the beginning, knowledgeable people recognized that taking the drug in this form could have results that were quite different from those that came from chewing coca leaves. Halstead certainly could have testified to this. Freud and Fleischl, too, no doubt. Cocaine hydrochloride is the form of the drug that was rediscovered by recreational users of cocaine in the late 1960s and early 1970s. Like their predecessors, they found that they could use it either by inhaling the powder through the nose or by injecting a liquid solution with a hypodermic syringe.

A few details are in order concerning the ways in which this salt of cocaine is used by recreational users of the drug. Inhalation of the powder, the process known as *snorting,* is normally done in one of two ways. Both of these ways often have a degree of ritual associated with them. It is often the case, for example, that the user rubs some of the drug onto his gums before inhaling the major portion of his dose. The procedure tends, for reasons that are discussed below, to prolong the effects of the drug. Rubbing the drug onto the gums also serves the purpose of using up the "residue" of the drug that is left over after snorting. Since it is really too bitter for him to enjoy by simply licking it up, he rubs it onto his gums where he tastes it less.

In one method of inhalation, the user employs a tiny spoon to scoop up an amount of drug suitable for inhaling. The spoonful of cocaine is carried to one nostril while the other nostril is held shut. Then with a rapid intake of breath the cocaine is inhaled into the nasal passage. In the second, more common method of snorting, the cocaine is spread out on a smooth surface, usually a surface made of glass, such as a mirror. A razor blade is used to arrange the cocaine into individual thin, parallel "lines" of drug, each line containing approximately 20–30 milligrams of drug. The user then inhales one or more of these lines, using a straw or a tightly rolled dollar bill to convey the cocaine to his nose. In some circles it was fashionable in the past to use a $100 dollar bill for this purpose. The conspicuous display of money in this way presumably gave testimony both to the high cost of the drug and to the ability of the provider to pay for it.

Injection of the drug requires the use of a hypodermic syringe and needle. The form of the drug injected is the same hydrochloride salt that is used when the drug is snorted. In the case of injection the drug is first dissolved in a suitable liquid such as water. The water solution of the drug is then placed in a syringe and injected. Typically, the injection is made directly into the bloodstream. The amount of cocaine injected in a single injection is about 16 milligrams.

It should be pointed out here that the injection of any drug places the user at additional risk. The risk is greater because of factors that are associated with the injection itself and are not specific to the particular drug injected. These are risk factors that go along with the intravenous (IV) injection of *any* drug. For example, most drugs sold on the street are not pure. They are typically adulterated ("cut") with other substances. Some of these added ingredients may produce effects that are more dangerous than those produced by the drug itself. In addition, many users share needles. This practice exposes them to any infections carried by others who share the same needle. In some American cities the major way in which AIDS is spread is through the use of shared needles. These additional complications of IV drug use will be explored more fully in the pages that follow.

How to Take a Good Thing and Make It Better

The isolation of cocaine from the coca plant changed forever the role that the drug would play in society. It is fairly easy to see why. First, the drug is pure cocaine. It is not mixed with other substances that take up space and do not contribute to the cocaine high. What you see is what you get. A gram of cocaine is a gram of cocaine. You don't have a half a pound of leaves and a lot of chewing to do in order to extract a small amount of the drug.

On the street, of course, there is always the possibility that a gram of cocaine does not really contain a gram of cocaine. In all probability it has been cut or adulterated by the supplier. He has added noncocaine ingredients to increase the apparent volume of the drug, and boost his profit margin. If the drug has been cut in this way, the user's problems are multiplied. The adulterants may cause him serious harm and may even kill him. Even if they do not, he has potentially serious problems relating to dose. If the concentration of cocaine varies from one purchase to another, it is quite easy to overdose without even knowing that such an outcome is possible.

But the basic reason that the pure drug has changed the cocaine scene has to do with the way in which the drug is taken. Unlike the case of the coca leaves chewed by the South American Indians, the pure drug is rarely taken orally. It is not ordinarily put into the digestive tract. This factor alone significantly increases the potency of the drug. The digestive system is not the most friendly environment for the drug. Millions of years of evolution have seen to that. As humans have evolved over the millennia, they have eaten many things that are harmful to them. (Try eating the wrong mushrooms, for example.) Over these same years, however, mechanisms have evolved which can counterbalance this oftentimes nondiscriminating palate. All of the blood, for example, that absorbs foodstuffs from the stomach and intestines goes immediately to the liver before it supplies the rest of the body. The liver, in turn, is the master organ of detoxification in the body. It does a good job of neutralizing many of the harmful substances that might be unwisely dumped into the digestive tract.

Inhalation of the pure drug gets cocaine into the blood stream and then into the brain (where it produces its most significant effects) without first going through the liver. A much larger portion of the drug that is inhaled gets to the brain before being detoxified than is the case when the drug is taken orally. This blood-brain relationship is crucial to an understanding of the effects of cocaine. It is also basic to an understanding of why crack is so much more devastating than cocaine hydrochloride.

The hypodermic syringe is important here, too. It allows the injection of the drug directly into the bloodstream. But, again, it is a purified drug which is injected, not crushed coca leaves. It is the availability of the pure drug that makes the hypodermic syringe so important.

So, the form of the drug is an important factor in understanding the effects that the drug produces. Would there not be a cocaine problem if pure cocaine did not exist? Would everything be all right if cocaine were available only in the form of coca leaves? The answer to this question is impossible to know. Cocaine users on the street would probably not willingly switch to chewing coca leaves. Nor would it be possible to do the controlled experiments necessary to answer the question. They would require the provision of cocaine in the two forms to large numbers of people, over a time period long enough (years) to compare their effects.

On the other hand, a minute's reflection suggests some parallels that lead to an appreciation of the importance of the form of the drug. When the Arabs introduced distillation into Europe, they changed drastically the pattern of alcohol consumption that was found there. Prior to this time the only alcoholic beverages that were available were naturally fermented products such as beer and wine. By its very nature natural fermentation can produce only products of low alcohol concentration. Distillation changed all that. Overnight European society made the transition from beverages containing, at a maximum, 12 percent alcohol to beverages containing 50 percent alcohol, with even higher concentrations easily obtainable with a little more effort. They thought highly of it, too. They named this new form of alcohol, in the various tongues spoken on the continent, "water of life."

Closer to the present day, the isolation of morphine from raw opium provides another example of the spiral of effects produced when purified and more concentrated forms of a drug become available. Pure morphine, again along with the hypodermic syringe, led to more widespread and more addictive patterns of narcotic use.

In this context, incidentally, it is interesting to note that heroin is simply morphine that has been heated in the presence of acetic acid, a maneuver that the drug czars have down pat. Heroin is not a legal medicine in the United States, whereas morphine is. In other words, heroin, the street drug, is simply a different *form* of the medical drug, morphine.

But all such interesting parallels aside, the important point is that pure cocaine produces tremendous dependence in the user. In this sense the form of the drug is a key factor in its abuse. The important question is, "How general is this relationship?" Or "Are there other forms of cocaine and, if so, do these also demonstrate that it is important to know the form of the drug if we are to understand how it produces its effects?"

There are two other forms in which cocaine is commonly seen on the street or in a recreational setting. These are *free-base* cocaine and the related form called *crack*. Free-base cocaine is obtained from cocaine hydrochloride by processes that, in a manner of speaking, reverse the process of extraction. The idea in producing free-base cocaine is to remove the hydrochloric acid from the salt form of the drug and liberate thereby the "natural" form of cocaine. This "natural" form is called a *base* by chemists and hence the liberated form is called a *free-base*. The user wants the free-base form of cocaine because, unlike the hydrochloride salt, it can be smoked. Smoking gets large amounts of cocaine into the system very quickly. So the euphoria achieved by using free-base cocaine is much more intense than is the high obtained by snorting the drug.

Free-basing cocaine has its hazards. To obtain the free base it is necessary to treat the cocaine powder with volatile solvents. The usual solvent has been ether. Ether, unfortunately, is highly explosive. It ignites at the slightest spark or flame. But the free base is destined to be smoked. This means that it is essential to remove all traces of the ether prior to lighting up. The comedian Richard Pryor learned the consequences of not doing so on the day his free-basing procedure went up in flames. He was badly burned.

Crack is essentially the product of a cheap and safe means of obtaining cocaine in smokable form, a form that has the desirable properties of a free base. The process involves treating cocaine hydrochloride with baking soda. It yields the small "rocks" of cocaine-containing substance called crack. These rocks can be smoked in a small pipe, and the resultant loading of the system with cocaine occurs with the rapidity and force of free-base cocaine.

Some of these facts about the various forms of cocaine are summarized in Table 3.1.

The problems associated with cocaine use have been much exacerbated by the introduction of free-base cocaine and crack. Both of these forms of cocaine are smoked, and smoking produces effects that seem to be even more intense than those produced by intravenous injection. Just as the IV user is carried higher and dropped lower than the user who snorts the drug, the smoker of crack attains peaks and reaches depths that are not frequently matched by the IV user. Smoking cocaine preparations guarantees that the maximum amount of drug will enter the body in the minimum time. The physiological reasons for this are examined in the next chapter.

The appearance of crack, especially, has fundamentally worsened society's cocaine problem. First, it is cheap. Just a few years ago, cocaine was quite expensive. It was available only in the crystalline form and at a very high price. Because of its price its use was associated with wealthy and glamorous segments of society. Some people even believed that the high price benefited society, arguing that the cocaine experience yielded such intense pleasure that everyone who used it would become addicted if it were not for the fact that the drug was so expensive.

Crack, however, has changed all that. Anyone can afford to buy it, even children. Much more significant, however, the rapidity and the intensity of its effects have introduced many people to a vicious cycle of boom and bust. For small amounts of money they can purchase a lightning trip to the heights of ecstasy. Small matter, it would seem, if every trip is followed by a fall into a depressive pit.

TABLE 3.1
RELATIONSHIPS AMONG VARIOUS FORMS OF COCAINE

Form of Cocaine	Typical Use	Time/Intensity		Addiction Risk
		Onset of effect	Intensity of effect	
Coca Leaves	Chewing	Slowest	Weakest	Lowest
Cocaine Hydrochloride	Snorting	3–5 minutes	Intense	High
Cocaine Hydrochloride	Intravenous	Immediate	Very intense	Very high
Cocaine Free Base	Smoking	Immediate	Very intense	Very high
Crack	Smoking	Immediate	Most intense	Highest

After all, all that is necessary to crawl out of the pit is another hit of crack, another toke on the pipe. And therein lies the snare of this form of cocaine. The highs are so high that they are followed by lows that are lower than low. And the only remedy, always as close at hand as your nearest drug dealer, is another hit of the drug.

But what do these highs represent? What has cocaine done to the body in order to bring all of this about? It is necessary to realize that no matter how the cocaine experience is described, no matter how personalized the reports of the users are, the cocaine experience is the result of specific physical changes in bodily processes that are produced by the drug. No drug produces magical, qualitative changes in our experienced world or in ourselves. No drug makes us better people. No drug can endow us with more desirable traits of personality or character. The most any drug can do is to bring about quantitative changes in the way in which the cells in our body work. Most of the mysticism and naivete that are such prominent aspects of the public debate on drug abuse would disappear if this fundamental truth were apprehended.

Chapter 4

What It's Like to "Do Cocaine"

> "Woe to you, my Princess, when I come I will kiss you quite red and feed you till you are plump—you shall see who is stronger, a gentle little girl who doesn't eat enough or a big wild man who has cocaine in his body. In my last severe depression I took coca again and a small dose lifted me to the heights in a wonderful fashion . . ."

No one has said it better. When Sigmund Freud wrote these lines to his fiancée, he epitomized what people are looking for when they turn to cocaine. It's all there in those few words, the good feelings, the feelings of mastery, the feelings of sexual prowess. While he may have been slower than most of his colleagues to appreciate the *hazards* of cocaine use, Freud zeroed in on the feel-good aspects of the drug with remarkable speed.

What had he found out? What have millions of cocaine users since then found out? How does cocaine make you feel? What kinds of feelings are these that make people come back again and again for more of the drug?

There are several ways in which this question can be pursued. One is to ask cocaine users what they feel like when they take the drug. When they take the drug they feel differently than they did before they took it. Many of these differences are due to changes in the way the drug user feels about himself. Freud certainly had a changed view of himself after taking cocaine. He felt better about himself. He was no longer depressed. Cocaine, in the short run at least, banished the feelings of sadness and disappointment that went along with a career that seemed to be stalled. He felt better about his physical abilities. He probably felt better about his ability as a lover. This is potent stuff. It is no wonder that he was eager to spread the good news about cocaine to his friends, associates, and family and to almost anyone else who would listen.

Testimony by Freud and other cocaine users has produced a catalog of effects that is useful in understanding the cocaine problem. While Freud's words lead to some pretty good guesses about cocaine's effect on his self-image, they do not get quite close enough to the nature of the cocaine experience. In particular, his remarks do not tell us anything about *how* the drug produces these changes in self-image.

Another approach is to investigate the effects of cocaine on the major organ systems of the body. The changes that cocaine produces in the individual's self-concept do not occur in a vacuum. Freud's good feelings about himself were the result of a number of physical alterations in body function that cocaine produces almost immediately after the drug is taken. These changed body functions very rapidly produce marked shifts in the way we experience our bodies and our minds. When people say that cocaine makes them feel good, they are really making a global judgment about how they experience these drug-produced alterations. If the cocaine problem is to be approached rationally, it is important to know more about how cocaine acts on the body.

Both approaches are taken in this chapter: the subjective reports of cocaine users and a description of the alterations produced by cocaine on the major organ systems of the body. Cocaine-induced alterations in one of these organ systems, the nervous system (and especially the brain), are singled out for special attention in the following two chapters. Why this special attention to the brain?

Because the alterations that cocaine produces in the brain's functions account for the powerful addicting character of the drug.

It's Like Art. I Might Not Know Much About It, but I Sure Know What I Like When I See It.

Making sense out of descriptions of the cocaine experience is not quite as easy as it sounds. If you talk to cocaine users and ask them what the drug does to them, you are liable to be surprised. They will report many different effects. You will find that the effects reported vary with the user and with the extent of his experience with cocaine. (Is he a first-time user or has he been using the drug regularly for a long time?) The effects will vary with his dose of the drug and with his method of taking it. (Is he snorting a few lines of the crystal a few times a month, or is he smoking crack every day?) Finally, the effects he reports will vary with the setting in which he takes the drug. (Is he taking the drug at a party where everyone is getting high? Is he a lonely individual shooting up in the isolation of a cheap hotel room?)

In spite of this variability, the major classes of cocaine effects can be described quite readily. Most of the reported effects involve changes in *mood,* changes in arousal level or *energy,* and changes related to an *altered awareness of bodily sensations.* Cocaine also produces modifications in one's perception of *sexual arousal.* These subjective reactions to cocaine are summarized in Table 4.1.

TABLE 4.1
THE EFFECTS OF COCAINE ON SELECTED PSYCHOLOGICAL
AND BEHAVIORAL RESPONSES

Reactions to Cocaine	Direction of Change	Evaluation of Change
Change in energy	Increase	Positive
Change in mood	Improvement	Positive
Change in bodily sensations	Increased awareness	Variable
Change in sexual interest	Increased or decreased depending on duration and amount of drug use	Generally positive but variable. Depends on several factors

Changes in Arousal or Energy Level

The experience most consistently described by users of the drug is a burst of energy. Many cocaine users report that the drug makes them feel as if their physical and mental powers have been increased. The user feels that anything is possible and that he is capable of accomplishing almost any task. Freud spoke of being "lifted to the heights" by the drug. Statements like the following are routinely reported:

"My mind seems to work better when I do cocaine."
"My thoughts are freed up. I concentrate better."
"My thoughts come more rapidly than usual."
"I can remember more things and the memories are sharper and clearer."

If you do cocaine, in other words, you are going to have some pretty satisfying thoughts running around in your head. You are going to be mentally alert like never before. You'll feel so "up," so much on top of things, that any of your shortcomings will seem like history. You say your abilities and talents aren't appreciated by your boss? What does he know? And what difference does it make, anyway? Cocaine has made *you* realize just how good you are!

You do the drug and your mind starts to race. It's awesome how you're able to capture images and ideas one after the other with a clarity that you've never known before. Your mental energy is almost overpowering. You find yourself coming up with solutions to problems that have been bugging you for as long as you can remember. Or at least this is the way things seem while cocaine is still playing with your mind. No wonder you feel so good! After all, you've got the energy and the mental equipment, you've got the smarts, to meet any challenge that the world might throw your way!

Inhalation of the drug begins to produce these effects almost always within three minutes. The maximum high or peak experience following snorting occurs after about 15 to 20 minutes. Most users report the effects have worn off after about 60 to 90 minutes. When the drug is injected intravenously, the onset of these and other effects is virtually instantaneous, with the peak experienced approximately 3 to 5 minutes after injection. Most people who inject the drug report that the effects have essentially worn off after about 30 to 40 minutes.

That there is a difference in the rapidity of the effects of the two methods of administration is significant. The intravenous user experiences effects that are much more intense than those experienced by the intranasal user. The experiences are so much more intense that they may have an added dimension to them. Because of the rapid onset of effects the IV user experiences an initial "rush" of intense sensation that has been described by some as "mind blowing" and by others as "better than sex." In addition, the effects wear off much more abruptly following IV use than following inhalation. In effect, the IV user is raised higher and dropped lower than is the user who inhales the drug.

Of course, as might be expected from the observations made at the end of the previous chapter, all such effects of cocaine are delivered with even greater rapidity and greater "clout" with free base or crack.

Changes in Mood

Mood changes are usually experienced and reported as increased feelings of well-being. The emotional tone of the cocaine user has changed, and in a positive direction. There is an emotionally satisfying aspect to the drug experience. The user's preoccupation with current difficulties is erased, troubles are forgotten, and he feels at peace with himself and the world.

"I don't feel discouraged like I usually do."
"I feel really relaxed."
"I wish this kind of contentment would never end."
"It's kind of like floating above it all."

You now not only realize how good you are, that you can do almost anything, but you *feel* great, too. Everything is cool, laid-back. The kicked-up mental energy and intellectual sharpness combined with this general sense of well-being has you feeling better than you've ever felt before. You might be elated and talking a lot. Nevertheless, even with the excitement that the drug has triggered, even with the edge that you now have, you experience a generalized sense of relaxation. You have a comforting kind of inner peace that you don't ordinarily run into during the day-to-day grind. This feeling of relaxation may seem to be a surprising effect from a drug that frequently makes people talkative and excited. Nonetheless, cocaine users commonly describe what the drug does for them in this way.

Altered Body Sensations

"I have this funny feeling in my stomach."
"I feel a little weird."

If you're doing cocaine, some of these feelings may upset you, at least for a brief period. If you're like most users, though, you'll probably be able to handle them. Like most users, you'll probably get used to these weird sensations. You'll probably end up by regarding them as a good part of the whole drug experience. You may even come to welcome these unpleasant sensations as reliable signals that the best is sure to come.

Cocaine and Sex

And now for one of the really big questions. What about cocaine and sex? Does cocaine make sex better? Does it make it more likely? Does cocaine increase sex drive? Does cocaine put new life into sexual relationships that are dulled and routine? Is cocaine really the aphrodisiac that much popular opinion has always held it to be?

The answers are not easy to come by. The effect of cocaine on sexuality is enormously complicated. Remember Helen and Charley. The role of cocaine in their sexual relations was not a simple one. The effect of the drug on their sexual activity changed over time. In the beginning, their sexual activities were enhanced by cocaine. In the end, the drug made sex seem trivial and boring by comparison. Incidentally, the change in their sexual behavior is related in an important way to an understanding of why cocaine is such an addicting drug. Cocaine was able to cause two normal, healthy young people to lose most of their interest in sex. In a later chapter I will point out how cocaine's action in the brain can produce this result.

One of the reasons that the relationship between cocaine and sex is so complicated is that human sexuality itself is enormously complicated. Sexual interactions are among the most exquisitely sensitive of all human interchange. A disturbance or a change in sexual behavior often signals a change in the overall quality of the relationship between partners. Sexual activity typically involves intimacy, openness and sharing. It has the potential to lay vulnerability on the line. As a consequence, sexual performance is often easily influenced by emotional or psychological difficulties. The experienced therapist knows that shifts of attitudes or changes in performance in the sexual area are often early warning signs of other trouble, often of a more profound nature, in other aspects of a relationship. Superimpose a powerful drug on this delicate state of affairs and all kinds of complications are possible.

The question of cocaine and sex is not at all a new one. The effect of the drug on sexual activity has been discussed and debated almost since the first reports of the coca plant in the sixteenth century. The plant has long been used as an aphrodisiac by natives in South America. In the United States no other drug, with the possible exception of amphetamine, has been so consistently associated in the popular imagination with sex. Even marijuana must take a back seat to cocaine in this regard. A consistent part of the folklore regarding cocaine is that it enhances both sexual arousal and sexual performance. Such a widely held belief merits attention. There just may be something to it.

The bottom line, though, is that there is no clear evidence that cocaine, *in and of itself,* functions as an aphrodisiac. There is no clear evidence that cocaine, the drug itself, serves either to increase sex drive or to enhance sexual performance.

Why, then, do reports abound that cocaine does increase sexuality? Why is it that Helen's description of the changes in her sexuality (and in Charley's, as well) is so commonly repeated in the reports of cocaine users? The major reason for this discrepancy between everyday reports and the position of many scientists is found in the scientist's reluctance to draw conclusions on the basis of uncontrolled, anecdotal data. The casual user of cocaine may be quite definite in telling you, "Hey, you bet it does! Coke is a real turn-on!" The scientist, however, being much more aware of the subtleties involved in matters of cause and effect, will demand a more rigorous standard of proof. While the reactions of the cocaine user in this area may be more relevant than the musings of the scientist, it would be a good idea to accord some space to scientific thinking on this point.

Several factors are at work here. Table 4.2 illustrates several ways in which cocaine use could be closely associated with increased sexual desire and increased sexual activity, even if the drug did not act *directly* to produce these increases.

Cocaine is a central nervous system stimulant. That is to say, it speeds up brain activity. This stimulating characteristic of the drug is what produces the increase in arousal level. People on cocaine are "up." They are more responsive to both their external environment and their internal state. They are also more aware of the effect of their own actions on other people. Sexual excitement, moreover, is a high arousal state that has much in common with the physiological arousal brought about by cocaine. When you're sexually aroused, you certainly are more attuned to the world around you (or at least to particular aspects of it). You are also more aware of your body's responses to that world.

This similarity between generalized central nervous system (CNS) arousal and sexual arousal suggests several means by which cocaine could bring about an increased interest in sexual activity. First it is possible that part of the general arousal pattern involves a direct stimulation of nerve pathways involved in the sexual response. That is, one of the components of the arousal and increased energy level caused by cocaine could be specific sexual arousal. If the drug did this, it would certainly qualify as an aphrodisiac.

Scientists point out, on the other hand, that the arousal produced by cocaine does not have to have a specific sexual component to it

TABLE 4.2
SOME POSSIBLE RELATIONSHIPS BETWEEN COCAINE AND SEXUAL AROUSAL

Suggested Reasons for Relationship	Proposed Mechanism
Central nervous system and autonomic nervous system stimulation	a. Direct sexual arousal b. General arousal c. Enhanced sensory responsiveness
Effects associated with setting in which drug is taken	a. Illegal activity b. Denial of prevailing moral code c. General relaxation of behavioral restraints

in order to produce increases in sexual responsiveness. There are at least two ways in which this could happen.

First, the increased arousal produced by the drug could have enough characteristics in common with sexual arousal that the person could confuse the two states. Sexual arousal, after all, is a multifaceted physiological state, involving complex CNS and autonomic nervous system responses. It could well be the case, in other words, that the increased arousal produced by cocaine is a nonspecific, general arousal that the individual may, under certain circumstances, *interpret* as increased sexual interest or stimulation.

Second, another suggestion is that cocaine increases sexual interest as a by-product of increased sensitivity to *all* aspects of the external environment. The theory is that cocaine enhances the effect of sensory stimulation in general, and that this may result in increased sexual interest and desire. The idea goes something like this: cocaine has special effects on the nerves that bring us information about what is going on in the world around us. Nerves that convey information about this world—what it looks like, what it smells like, what it feels like, what it tastes like—are pushed into a hyper-responsive state by the drug. In this state of increased responsivity, they lead to an accentuation or exaggeration of incoming messages about what is going on in the surrounding environment. Sounds may take on new and sharper meaning. The sense of smell may be more acute. Things may be seen more clearly. Sexual interest and responsiveness may be increased because the nerves that respond to sexual stimulation are more active. Or they may be more finely tuned and more disposed to respond to objects and events of potential sexual significance. Many cocaine users report that cocaine, at least in the short run, does indeed have this effect. (A similar effect is often attributed to amphetamine, another powerful central nervous system stimulant.)

But all of this is highly theoretical. Of more immediate interest are cocaine users' reports of actual associations between cocaine and specific sexual responses. These comments suggest a direct link between cocaine and increased sexual arousal. Such reports, as well as some similar findings from clinical research, reveal several important things.

• Cocaine can lead to increased erections in males.

- Some of the erections apparently last for unusually long periods.
- Cocaine can inhibit and retard orgasm in both males and females.

Do these reports suggest that cocaine does indeed produce an increase in sexual pleasure? There is some ambiguity here. Retarded orgasm may be regarded as either a desirable or an undesirable effect. (Patients taking some of the medications used to treat mental illness often *complain* about just this effect of the drugs.) Consequently, the drug that produces this effect may be regarded as enhancing or diminishing sex. Is retarded orgasm regarded as increased ("better") performance? In males, especially, are prolonged erections and retarded orgasms taken as evidence of increased sexual prowess, or is the retarded orgasm regarded as a "failure," a negative sexual consequence of using the drug?

The drug has also been used in a sexual context by direct application to the sexual organs of both males and females. If the drug is applied directly to the genitals, a tingling sensation occurs and the length of intercourse is said to be increased. A tingling like this may be easily interpreted as evidence of sexual arousal. If so, the drug may appear to have aphrodisiac qualities. But it must be remembered that cocaine is a local anesthetic. The anesthetic effect of the drug on genital membranes may reduce the sensation transmitted by nerves carrying sexual information. Under these conditions it would be possible to increase the duration of intercourse without any increase in pleasure.

Many authorities, in fact, feel that any enhancement that cocaine brings to human sexuality is not a direct effect of the drug at all. They agree that there are many cases where cocaine use leads to increases in sexual activity and enjoyment. People may, in fact, use cocaine to increase the quality, or at least the frequency, of sex in their lives. These authorities suggest, however, that the drug itself does not produce these effects. According to this view, increases in sexual activity associated with cocaine are more than likely due, as in the case of marijuana, to the expectations of the drug taker. The user of cocaine may actually experience an increase in sex drive. But this is because, consciously or unconsciously, he expects that the drug will have this effect. He is primed, in other words, to interpret the real changes the drug produces in his body as increases in sex interest or sex drive.

These authorities suggest, in addition, that the use of cocaine is usually accompanied by a loosening of the normal day-to-day constraints that modulate our behavior. Drug use, after all, is officially condemned by society. It is illegal. The use of drugs like cocaine is, implicitly, a denial of the prevailing moral code. Cocaine, these authorities say, may be associated with a sexual turn-on because it occurs in a situation where behavioral restraints, in general, have been tossed aside.

Here is a brief summary of the current thinking on the relationship between cocaine and sex:

- There are reasons to suspect that cocaine *could* act as an aphrodisiac. It leads to high-arousal states that are similar in many ways to sexual arousal.
- It is possible that part of the increased arousal involves nerve pathways that are involved in sexual stimulation.
- Cocaine may push all sensory processes, including the processing of sexual stimuli, into a hyperresponsive state.
- There are frequent reports associating cocaine with altered sexual performance, such as increased erection in males and delayed and more intense orgasm in both males and females.
- It is possible that all such effects are secondary to a change in outlook or expectation on the part of the user.

All of these considerations have led one psychological investigator in this area to remark, "Does *any* substance qualify as a 'true' aphrodisiac? By God, if it walks like a horse and talks like a horse, let's call it a horse!"

I've Got You Under My Skin

One other effect of cocaine must be discussed at this point. Since Fleishl's time it has been known that cocaine is capable of producing psychosis under some circumstances. Psychosis entails having hallucinations and delusions. These kinds of behaviors are among the possible toxic reactions to the drug. A close look at some of the symptoms of *cocaine psychosis* will provide a better understanding of the range of effects that it produces. In addition, since these toxic reactions involve psychosis, they must be due to the action of the drug on the brain. An examination of these conditions can help to focus attention on the forthcoming discussion of cocaine's effect on the human brain.

A cocaine psychosis is serious business. Just how serious is evident when one remembers what the psychologist or psychiatrist means by the word "psychosis." These mental health professionals use this word to refer, roughly, to mental conditions that the legal profession refers to as insanity. A psychosis is a disturbed mental condition that may be severe enough to require that the afflicted individual be admitted to a mental hospital. Cocaine is capable of deranging the brain's chemistry to such an extent that people are no longer rational, no longer capable of directing their own affairs. Their minds and their behaviors are disorganized to the point that they may be a danger to themselves and to other people.

What are the symptoms of this kind and degree of extreme mental breakdown? The symptoms are remarkably similar in many ways to those shown by patients suffering from *paranoid schizophrenia,* a serious form of mental illness. The symptoms include delusions and hallucinations. Delusions are firmly held but outlandishly erroneous belief systems. Paranoid delusions, the most common type, are fantastic beliefs that one is being persecuted or that one is an especially important, even exalted, person. Paranoid delusions may convince the individual that he is being spied upon by the CIA, that his tormentors are manipulating his thoughts with unseen laser radiations, and that all of these things are happening because he is a very important person.

Hallucinations are realistic perceptions of people or objects outside of the person that occur when those people or objects are not really present. The hallucinating person may *see* things that are not there. In this case he would be said to suffer from *visual* hallucinations. He may *hear* the voices of people who are not present. They may talk to him or about him. He would be experiencing *auditory* hallucinations. He may even feel people, insects or animals touching his body when no such event is taking place. In this case he would be experiencing *tactile* hallucinations.

In cocaine psychosis any of these types of mental derangements may be observed. The individual may appear quite delusional, believing himself surrounded by others who are plotting against him. The nature of the delusion, the specific type of plot, will vary from individual to individual, but the delusional nature of the belief system is easily seen in each case. The hallucinations usually associated with cocaine psychosis, on the other hand, frequently are quite similar from one individual to another. These hallucinations usually consist of sensations that bugs are crawling over, or frequently under, the skin. The psychologist's term for the experience is *formication,* a term derived from the Latin *formica,* meaning ant. Frequently, heavy cocaine users who have experienced this type of hallucination have markedly ulcerated locations on their skin. In these cases there may be many small lesions scattered over the surface of the skin, including the areas around the eyebrows and the hairline. These lesions are the scars remaining from repeated attempts to dig imaginary insects from under the skin with the point of a knife or other sharp instrument.

In most cases of cocaine psychosis, the mental impairment diminishes as the drug is metabolized and clears the body. As the body does its normal work of ridding itself of toxic substances, the level of cocaine is reduced. As the level falls, so, normally, do the symptoms decrease in severity and disappear.

All Anyone Is Looking For in This Life Is a Sympathetic Response

How does cocaine bring about these rapid changes? How are these changed perceptions of the body and of the outside world related to the effects of cocaine on the various organs of the body? For, in the final analysis, it is the effect of cocaine on these organs that is the basis for all of the cocaine users' reports, no matter how varied.

There are two broad classes of cocaine actions on body organs and tissues. On the one hand, there are those actions that occur in the brain, a part of the central nervous system (CNS). On the other hand, there are those actions of the drug that take place in portions of the body outside of the CNS. These are referred to as *peripheral* actions of the drug.

When discussing the reports of cocaine users we were concerned with the *effects* of the drug. In the present context, when talking about the direct interaction between cocaine and body tissues we want to focus attention on the *action* of the drug. This distinction between action and effect is important. The effects that the drug produces, including the effects that the user reports, are the result of specific physical or chemical actions of the drug on his body tissues and organs.

Much of the mystique surrounding cocaine and all other drugs disappears when this basic fact is recognized. All of the effects drugs produce can be boiled down to the result of actions of the drugs on specific organs and tissues in the body, actions that, in principle, are easily understood. There is no magic, no pharmacological sleight-of-hand, no keys to inner truth or inner peace. Drugs are not a royal road to creativity. They produce, pure and simple, direct chemical disruption of the normal work of selected cells and organs.

Effects on the Sympathetic Nervous System

Think about the last time you were afraid. *Really* afraid. Don't worry too much about what it was that made you afraid. Concentrate on what it *felt* like. Try to remember the shortness of breath, the way you seemed to be taking in air in little gasps, because of the tightness in your chest. Remember your heart beating with a force that threatened to break right through your rib cage. Remember the way your eyes were opened so wide that it seemed as if invisible fingers were pulling back your eye lids so that you wouldn't miss anything that happened around you. And your gut, the tightness, the scrunching down, the feeling that all of your abdominal muscles had been contracted into a solid wall. The large muscles of your arms, legs and shoulders were similarly contracted. You were energized, prepared to repel the forces that were threatening to overcome you.

If you can remember such a time in your life, and if you can remember the way you felt, you are remembering what it's like to be dominated by a highly aroused *sympathetic nervous system,* the portion of your nervous system that takes over when you are frightened. It also takes over when you feel that you are threatened and must fight for your survival. For these reasons, the pattern of responses that you've just remembered are referred to as a *fight-or-*

flight response. It is a response so basic to survival that it has been around for millions of years of evolution in all mammalian species. You have it. Your dog has it. Laboratory rats have it. It's important to understand this response of the sympathetic nervous system (SNS) because cocaine produces a response that is very much the same as the fight-or-flight response.

The sympathetic nervous system is one of two branches of the human *autonomic nervous system* (ANS). The other branch is called the *parasympathetic nervous system* (PNS). The ANS controls the activity of those muscles and glands that are usually thought of as involuntary, the rate at which your heart beats, for example. Blood pressure is regulated by ANS control over the size of the blood vessels. The secretion of digestive juices and the rate of movement of food through the digestive tract, the passage of air through the lungs and bronchial tubes, the elimination of feces and urine, and the state of excitation of your sexual organs are among the many aspects of the "internal environment" that are controlled in large part by autonomic nervous system activity.

Of course, you're not in a state of fear most of the time. This is because the two branches of the ANS operate in a kind of mutual opposition that keeps the internal environment more or less in a state of balance. Deviations from this balance represent well-regulated and temporary departures in favor of domination by either the sympathetic or the parasympathetic branch. If one is fearful or aroused, the sympathetic branch dominates. Heart rate is increased; more air is taken in through the lungs; blood is routed to the large skeletal muscles and away from the digestive system; the pupils of the eyes dilate, and the aroused individual is prepared for action.

When you are relaxed, parasympathetic activity predominates. Heart rate decreases; intake of oxygen goes down; blood flow is increased to the digestive tract, facilitating the work of these organs; the pupils contract because of lessened interest in processing information from the environment. The parasympathetically dominated person is less prepared for immediate action.

Drugs are potent disturbers of this natural order of things. Many drugs bring about a radical shift in favor of one branch of the ANS over the other. Cocaine is one such drug. Cocaine is referred to by the pharmacologist as a *sympathomimetic* drug because it mimics overactivity of the sympathetic nervous system. Cocaine causes the body to undergo a pattern of ANS changes that would normally be seen only when the sympathetic nervous system has established dominance over the parasympathetic system. The drug produces a sympathetic response that is characteristic of high arousal states such as fear.

Why, then, doesn't the cocaine user become fearful in the face of this sympathetic dominance? Simply because he or she knows that the changes being experienced are drug-induced, and that pleasant rather than unpleasant things are about to occur. The increased sympathetic arousal is worked into and interpreted as a part of an expected well-being and euphoria. At times, however, the drug experience can get out of hand and the user is engulfed with feelings of anxiety or even terror. He or she looses sight of the fact that the bodily changes being experienced are drug-related. The drug user is overwhelmed by feelings and bodily sensations that can easily be recognized as fear. The result is panic and at times a disintegration of personality to the point of a toxic psychosis.

Effects on the Cardiovascular System

Among the most prominent effects of cocaine are those that produce changes in the functioning of the heart and blood vessels. Some of these effects are indirect, the result of cocaine's actions in the brain, while others are due to direct effects of the drug on the organs themselves. The major direction of all of these effects is to stimulate the cardiovascular system. Heart rate is increased. Blood pressure is increased. The drug produces a dramatic rise in blood pressure, due both to actions in the brain and in the peripheral system.

One of the direct effects of cocaine can kill you very quickly, even before you have a chance to respond. Cocaine can cause cardiac arrest as a result of several different actions on the heart. Acute myocardial infarction (the death of cardiac muscle) may occur as a result of drug-induced spasm of the coronary arteries or as a consequence of drug-induced coronary thrombosis. Additionally, serious cardiac arrhythmias (irregular heartbeats) can occur as a result of cocaine's ability to increase the stimulation of cardiac muscle by the sympathetic nervous system. There is no known way to predict these outcomes. They have occurred in experienced users taking large amounts of the drug as well as in first-time users taking low doses.

Effects on Body Temperature

Cocaine leads to increases in body temperature that are sometimes quite dramatic. The effect is due to increased heat production and to decreased heat lost. Cocaine may cause the body to produce more heat because the drug usually produces an increase in activity level. The drug also reduces the body's ability to get rid of excess heat. This effect occurs because the drug constricts the blood vessels in the skin. When these blood vessels are constricted, the body is unable to get rid of the increased heat.

Cocaine also exerts a direct effect on the brain's temperature regulating centers, producing, in severe cases, the so-called cocaine fever that is a prominent feature of cocaine poisoning.

Effects on the Central Nervous System

Cocaine is a stimulant drug. It has an excitatory effect on nerve cells in the brain. Cocaine, in fact, is the most potent of all of the drugs that are known to stimulate the brain. This action in the brain causes nerve cells to increase their activity, which in turn produces the increased activity, the heightened talkativeness, the restlessness and the increased excitement that are characteristic of the cocaine experience. So it is that users routinely speak of being able to party for forty-eight or seventy-two hours without experiencing any need to sleep.

The stimulation of the brain by cocaine is a dose-related phenomenon. Relatively low doses produce the kind of excitement just described. If the dose is increased enough, the additional burden of stimulation imposed on brain cells may be too much for them to bear. They may be overstimulated to the point where they may not be able to keep up with the demands of the drug. In this case they will give up. They will shut down and stop working. When this happens, the brain moves rapidly from a highly stimulated condition to a depressed condition. Under these conditions, it is very likely that among the nerve cells that quit working are those that are immediately essential to maintaining life. For example, nerve cells that are responsible for maintaining normal patterns of breathing may cease to function. You stop breathing and you die.

The Shortest Distance Between Two Points Is the Bloodstream

How can one drug produce such a variety of changes in so many different organs and tissues? Moreover, when you snort the drug, how does it come to influence so many different parts of the body, most of them located quite some distance from the nose, the point of entry into the body? These are some basic questions in pharmacology, questions that should be asked about any drug. The answers are fundamental. They are the same for any drug, from the penicillin that the physician prescribes to the crack that is sold illegally on the street.

The best way to find these answers is to trace the route cocaine follows from the point it enters the body to the organs that it attacks. Following the drug in this way will also provide an understanding of why crack is a more dangerous form of the drug than is the crystalline salt, and why it is better able to dominate the life of the user.

For the most part, drugs act at specific sites, and in specific ways, within the body. As an example, consider antibiotics. These drugs are extremely effective in curing bacterial infections. A wide variety of antibiotics has been developed since the introduction of penicillin in the 1940s. One reason for the continued development of new antibiotics is that they differ significantly in their effectiveness against various species of bacteria. This difference in effectiveness, in turn, is related to the fact that different antibiotics kill bacteria by different means. Some antibiotics, such as pencillin, kill bacteria by preventing them from maintaining the rigid cell wall that is necessary to their survival. Other antibiotics, such as erythromycin, destroy bacteria by inhibiting the bacteria from manufacturing essential proteins. Still other antibiotics, such as bacitracin, kill bacteria by destroying the protective functions of the bacterial cell membrane. The point is that different drugs may bring about the desired control of bacterial infection by quite different means. The *effect* of the drugs, in this case the destruction of bacteria, can be the result of several different *actions* of the drugs (cell wall breakdown, interference with metabolism, etc.). Different drugs can bring about a given effect by acting in various ways throughout the body. In the pharmacologist's terminology, drugs have different *sites* and *mechanisms of action.*

The second important point to keep in mind is that drugs commonly gain entrance to the body at locations that are quite far from their sites of action. If a patient is suffering from the type of accumulation of fluid in the lungs called pneumonia, the physician may treat this condition by administering antibiotics orally or intramuscularly. In both cases the drug is introduced into the body (in the stomach, say, or in the muscles of the buttocks) at some distance from the lungs. How does it get from the entry point, the site of administration, to the point in the body where it is needed? The vehicle, or means of transportation, that carries the drug from its site of administration to its site of action is the bloodstream. The orally administered drug, like the drug administered by injection, ultimately destroys the bacteria because it is carried to the site of battle by the bloodstream. If the drug is to do its work it must be *absorbed* into the bloodstream and *distributed* to its site of action. If the drug cannot get to its site of action, it will not be able to produce its effect. Some cases of bacterial infection of the brain, for example, are very difficult to treat because it is difficult for some antibiotics to gain entry to the brain from the bloodstream.

Cocaine and Crack: Fast and Faster

What all of this means is that the speed at which a drug is absorbed is a major determinant of the intensity of the response to the drug. The blood rapidly circulates around the body. Once a drug has gained access to the circulatory system, distribution throughout the body occurs quickly. Hence, the most important factor affecting the time between the administration of a drug and the appearance of its effects is the speed of absorption into the circulatory system. Factors that hasten this absorption will intensify the peak effects of the drug.

There are several variables that affect the rate of absorption of drugs, including the structure of the drug and the acidity of the body tissues where the drug is introduced. In the majority of cases, however, the most important factor governing rate of absorption is simply the extent of the blood supply at the place where the drug is introduced into the body. The rule is simple: the better the blood supply, the more rapid the absorption; the more rapid the absorption, the greater the peak effect. It is this factor of differences in the blood supply at the place where the drug enters the body that accounts for the greater intensity of response when crack is smoked compared to the response intensity when the crystalline form of the drug is snorted.

When cocaine is snorted, the chemical lodges in the mucous linings of the nasal passages. These are moist tissue layers, and placing the drug there is equivalent to dissolving it in a water solution. Indeed, this dissolving of the chemical is the essential first step in the absorption of the drug. Only after the drug is dissolved is it capable of passing across the layers of tissue that make up the lining of the nasal cavities. The drug thus gains access to the bloodstream, which is on the other side of these tissues. This entire process of dissolving and moving across tissue layers takes time.

Additional time is required before significant levels of cocaine build up in the bloodstream. There are two reasons for this. One, the nasal cavity is a small space, and the volume of blood supplied to its small interior surface area is not large. Hence, the area of interface between the drug "on the outside" and the blood supply "on the inside" is not a large one. The drug, in the process of gaining access to the bloodstream, is effectively held up at the entry portal, the absorbing surface of the nasal cavity.

There is another factor that slows down the entry of cocaine into the bloodstream when it is taken intranasally. Cocaine is a potent vasoconstrictor, which means that it reduces the flow of blood through the blood vessels in the nose. Ironically, the very presence of the drug contributes to the delay in its gaining access to the blood supply.

Consider, by contrast, the situation when crack is smoked. In this case the cocaine is contained in the smoke that is delivered to the lungs. The lungs are specialized organs whose primary function is to exchange substances between the air inhaled and the bloodstream. This is how oxygen in the air is exchanged for carbon dioxide in the blood. This process is extremely efficient because of the structure of the lung, which possesses a great blood supply in its vast network of capillaries. These capillaries, furthermore, are spread out over a vary large surface area in such a way that the bloodstream is separated from the inhaled air by only one cell membrane. The system is designed to promote maximum interchange between the air and the bloodstream. Cocaine molecules, in the smoke from the crack, take advantage of this specialized exchange mechanism to enter the bloodstream rapidly and in huge amounts. In fact, the rate of cocaine entry into the blood by this route is almost as rapid as it is when injected directly into the veins. The result is peak cocaine effects that exceed by far those that are experienced when the drug is snorted. In this way the crack smoker experiences "highs" that are not easily attained by the user who snorts the drug.

Cocaine, at this point in the story, should no longer be a mysterious, enigmatic drug. What is not yet apparent, however, is *why* cocaine should be such an addictive drug. The answer to this question depends upon filling in one more piece of the puzzle. What remains to be discovered are the subtle biological strategies that cocaine employs when it reaches its target cells. To understand addiction we need to examine the ways in which cocaine disrupts the normal function of these cells. The following two chapters explore how cocaine works on its most important target, the human brain.

Chapter 5

Pleasure, Pleasure and More Pleasure: Cocaine, the Brain and Addiction

The Pleasure Connection

In 1954 Dr. James Olds, an experimental psychologist, made a fundamental discovery. He had placed tiny electrodes deep within the brains of his laboratory rats. By passing a minute electrical current through these electrodes, Olds was able to get his rats to perform any task that he chose. The rats seemed to work at the specified task because they liked the stimulation the scientist delivered to their brains. Although Olds's discovery was hailed as ground breaking, its connection with cocaine was not suspected. It was not at all apparent at the time that his discovery would one day help us understand how cocaine exercises its strong control over the addict.

Olds's work bears examining in some detail. If it were not for

James Olds's rats, knowledge about the addicting properties of cocaine would be in roughly the stage of development that it was at the time of Freud's infatuation with the drug. Just what, then, do rats with electrical probes in their brains have to do with cocaine?

Plenty.

The key to the relationship between Olds's rats and cocaine is simply that Olds's rats *liked* the stimulation that the scientist provided through the electrodes. Whenever the rats performed correctly, such as by pressing a lever when a signal light was flashed in their cage, the scientist delivered an electrical pulse to their brains. The stimulation was used to teach them the task and to keep them performing at a high level. They liked what Dr. Olds was doing to their brains. This is why they worked at the various tasks that Olds set for them, because their efforts led to more brain stimulation. Moreover, in the years since this initial discovery, it has become apparent that the rats liked the stimulation in a way closely related to the way in which the cocaine user likes cocaine.

The importance of Olds's discovery does not, however, lie simply in the fact that he found something that his rats liked. He found something much more important. What he found, it is now known, is the touchstone to why we, humans, enjoy or take pleasure in a whole range of things. Olds's discovery opened the door to an understanding of why people are able to experience pleasure at all. His experiments pointed the way to an understanding of the fact that the experience of pleasure is a direct consequence of the way in which the brain is organized.

Many things in life provide us with pleasure. Things like a good meal, for instance, or the satisfaction that comes from achievement, the smile of an approving mother, the caress of a lover, the ecstasy of sexual orgasm. It was not until Olds's discovery, however, that scientists began to unravel the things that these various events have in common. Olds's findings led to intensive efforts to understand the role of the brain in producing these feelings of pleasure. As a result of these efforts, it is now known that the intensely pleasurable feelings produced by cocaine are the result of the drug's ability to stimulate the brain directly, just as Olds's electrical currents did. Cocaine stimulates those areas in the brain that normally are involved in the experiencing of pleasure from a wide variety of sources.

There is irony in the fact that Olds's discoveries laid the groundwork for our current understanding of pleasure. At the time of his initial experiment he was not interested in pleasure. He was interested in displeasure. He was searching for those areas of the brain that inform us that something is *not* enjoyable.

A closer look at the procedures that he used will lead to an enhanced appreciation of the significance of what he found. In order to find areas of displeasure, he placed tiny electrodes in the brains of rats. He then passed a very small current through these electrodes in an attempt to see if it had a negative effect on the animal. A negative effect might be seen, for example, if the electrical stimulation caused an animal to react with signs of irritation or displeasure. Even better evidence that the stimulation had an unpleasant effect would be if the electrical current prevented the animal from doing something that it obviously liked to do. Thus, stimulation that caused a hungry animal to turn away from food, or a thirsty animal to turn away from water, could be considered to be unpleasant. Olds wanted to locate areas of the brain where stimulation produced negative effects. He found, instead, areas where the current had positive effects. He had located what have since come to be called *reward centers* of the brain.

Olds's discovery is a beautiful example of the dictum that "chance favors the prepared mind." Quite by accident, the electrode in one of the rats was placed in the wrong area of the brain. This animal, as a consequence, did not act as Olds expected. It did not react negatively to the stimulating current. Olds was astute enough to observe, however, that it was not simply a matter that the stimulation was without *any* effect on the animal. He noticed, rather, that the animal actually seemed to *like* the stimulation. The rat seemed to be looking for more of it. For example, it kept returning to the area of the cage where the stimulation was delivered. Olds correctly guessed the the animal was actually looking for additional stimulation. Subsequent experiments confirmed that this was indeed the case.

Since Olds's initial discovery, several areas of the brain have been found where stimulation has strong positive effects. These areas are sometimes referred to as *pleasure centers* because of early observations that animals like rats seemed to like being stimulated there. The psychologist calls these centers reward areas because stimulation applied here can effectively control the rat's behavior. The stimulation, in other words, is a reward.

Daily experience provides ample evidence that rewards are powerful tools for controlling behavior. Parents routinely reward their children when they act in the desired manner. The rewards may be words of praise, smiles, special treats, or other things that children want. People want many things and therefore many things can act as rewards, things such as food, money and sex. The significant thing about all such rewards is that people want them. They will work to obtain them. Or, to put it another way, an individual's behavior can be influenced and ultimately controlled by rewarding him appropriately. Direct stimulation of the reward areas of the brain, of the type carried out by Olds, is also able to exert this kind of influence or control over the animal. The rats in Olds's experiments would learn to perform any task that they were capable of performing when the only payoff to them was electrical stimulation of their brains.

But there is more to it than that. There is something about brain stimulation that makes it different from all other rewards. It is more powerful. Animals prefer it to other, more conventional rewards. A hungry rat will ignore food in order to work for brain stimulation, so diligently and constantly, in fact, that he will ignore the food that is available to him. He will starve to death in his quest for this reward.

There is even more to the story. An animal with electrodes in his brain will administer the stimulation to himself. The situation can be so arranged that when the animal presses a lever in his cage he causes the stimulation to be delivered to his brain. He easily learns that this is the case and will press the lever repeatedly and at a very high rate. If a rat is given an opportunity to do this, he will ignore food, water and sex and continue to press the lever until he is physically exhausted. The rat in this situation acts as if he were saying to you, "I know that there are other things in my surroundings that are interesting and enjoyable. I know that other rats are interested in them, and I was at one time myself. But now that you've introduced me to *this*, I no longer have the interest in those other things that I once did."

If brain stimulation is all that pleasurable for a rat, it is equally pleasurable for people? Don't we have here the key to relieving depression? Wouldn't this be a perfect way to banish the common feelings of unhappiness that most of us experience from time to time? Couldn't a lot of unhappy people be made to feel better simply by implanting electrodes in their brains? Think about the possibilities. Why go through periods when you're feeling kind of "down?" If you had a tiny electrode planted in your brain, you could overcome these feelings simply by giving yourself a little electrical jolt in your reward center.

As a matter of fact, similar things have been tried with humans in a limited number of cases. Electrodes *have* been implanted in human brains. The results are entirely consistent with what you would have expected. Stimulation of human reward centers is pleasurable. However, the idea has not caught on widely. Most of us are not comfortable with the kind of control that these procedures suggest. They contain a hint of Big Brother. Putting electrodes in the heads of human beings in order to control them seems to be taking too large a step in the direction of destroying individual liberty.

But what if results like these could be achieved without the surgery? What if the electrodes were not needed? What if it could be done with drugs?

If you're thinking along these lines, you have just penetrated to the hearts of Olds's discovery. There are important similarities between the behavior of Olds's rats and the behavior of the cocaine addict. The brain stimulation monopolized the interest of the rats. Brain stimulation diverted their attention from other significant aspects of their environment. They spent enormous amounts of time near the lever, which, when pressed, delivered the desired current to their brains. They pressed the lever thousands of times per hour, never seeming to tire of the stimulation that it provided. It even looked as if the effect of the stimulation was cumulative. The more the animal stimulated himself, the more stimulation he wanted. The animal that had been introduced to brain stimulation behaved as if it had discovered an entirely new dimension to its existence. It was as if this new experience had made most of the animal's other activities pale and insignificant in comparison.

Some of the cocaine addict's behaviors can be described in terms very similar to those used to describe Olds's rats. Cocaine addicts, too, have discovered a new dimension to their existence. They, too, have found a source of pleasure that causes them to lose interest in

other aspects of their lives. Remember that Helen and Charley virtually gave up sex when they became deeply involved with cocaine.
Cocaine addicts devote an enormous amount of time to drug-related
activities. Like Olds's rats, they administer this new type of stimulation over and over again. Finally, the very action of taking the drug
seems to make cocaine addicts want to take more of it.

These similarities hold the key to an understanding of the addictive power of cocaine. This is why a rational approach to cocaine
requires a closer look at the brain's pleasure centers.

Seeing, Talking, Feeling, Sex: Let's Get Organized

The discovery that the brain has specific centers for pleasure is
relatively new. It is, however, consistent with most of what has been
known about brain organization for over a hundred years. One fundamental idea holds that the brain, while always working as a
whole, is organized in such a way that some behaviors are highly
dependent on specific brain areas. Other, dissimilar behaviors are
highly dependent on other brain areas. Over the course of evolution
certain regions of the brain have become specialized to organize and
direct specific types of behavior.

Most of us are aware of this kind of localization of function in the
brain. We know that certain behaviors are dependent on specific
parts of the brain. Many of us have seen relatives or friends suffer
from stroke. Frequently the victim has been left with an inability to
speak. Except for this loss of speech, the patient's recovery may be
complete. He is able to leave the hospital and return home. He is
able to care for himself on a day-to-day basis. His mind works well,
and his personality is intact. He's the same person that we knew
before the illness. That is, the stroke has left him alive and relatively well, except that he is unable to speak. In these cases, the
stroke has destroyed the *speech center* of the brain, a part of the
brain known as *Broca's Speech Area* (see Figure 5.1). Similar
observations may be made in the case of a stroke that is limited to
paralyzing a limb or perhaps one side of the body. It is possible to
observe all of these deficits in people who are otherwise normal.
They have suffered specific losses in their abilities as a result of
damage to specific parts of the brain.

Other examples that come readily to mind show that particular

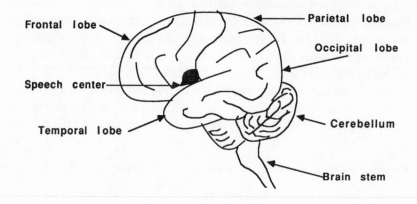

Fig. 5.1 The lobes of the cerebral hemispheres, showing the location of Broca's speech center

functions may depend heavily on the correct working of particular brain areas. An otherwise normal individual will be unable to see if a portion of the brain known as the visual cortex is destroyed. Some people with damage to different brain areas cannot smell. Others cannot taste. Still others cannot hear. In each of these cases a particular behavior is related to a specific portion of the brain.

What may not be so well recognized in these last examples, however, is that some very fundamental *experiences* depend on specific areas of the brain. The blind person has lost the *experience* of sight; the person who cannot smell has lost the *experience* of smell. Olds's discovery of reward centers in the brain is basic to an understanding of cocaine addiction because it demonstrates that the *experience* of pleasure is dependent upon specific brain areas.

This notion that the experience of pleasure depends upon specific brain events is fundamental, and provides the key to understanding how cocaine produces addiction. The idea is so basic, in fact, that it will be useful to look at one other example illustrating the relationship between the working of the brain and the experience of pleasure. This example is of sexual pleasure. It gets very close to the type of experience that cocaine provides to the user of the drug.

Sexual pleasure is, of course, one of the most intense of human experiences. The very intensity of this pleasure insures that people will seek out opportunities for sexual activity. The evolutionary significance of the pleasure to be found in sex is very easy to see. The inborn sexual drive insures that children will be produced and that the species will be propagated. What is perhaps not so easy to see is that the experience of sexual pleasure, like the experience of sights and sounds, depends on an intact and functioning brain. In a very real sense, when it comes to sex, it's all in your head.

Here's how the process works. During sexual activity, stimulation of the genitals causes nerves to carry information to the brain, informing it that such activity is taking place. When sexual activity occurs, the brain *interprets* what is going on as pleasurable. The brain transforms the messages carried by the nerves into a *perception* of pleasure. The experience of sexual pleasure requires the participation of the brain.

A few examples will illustrate this relationship. If a man has suffered injury to the spinal cord so that the nerves connecting the sexual organs to the brain have been severed, the experience of sexual pleasure will be markedly altered. For one thing, the genitals will no longer be capable of responding with sexual arousal to the sights, sounds and ideas that aroused him before the injury. Stimuli like erotic images, or the soft, entreating voice of a lover will be incapable of producing the arousal that they once did. All of the sights and sounds are recognized by the brain, but none of the information that the brain has processed will be translated into sexual excitement. There will be no erection, because the nerves that should convey the brain's experience of erotic stimulation can no longer carry the message to the sexual organs.

Notice that it is the brain that is the source of sexual arousal in this case. It is important to appreciate there is nothing wrong with our patient's sexual organs. Indeed, if the sexual organs are stimulated directly, he is capable of achieving and maintaining an erection. This is possible for him because intact, local spinal cord connections are sufficient to produce an erection. He can even be brought to ejaculation in this way. But the ejaculation is not appreciated by the patient as sexual pleasure. That is, he has no *experience* of climax or orgasm. Because of the severed nerves, the stimulation of the genitals has not been able to reach the brain, and he experiences no sexual pleasure from the manipulation of the sex organs. Interestingly enough, the same man might be able to experience the intense pleasure of sexual orgasm under the right circumstances. He may be capable of experiencing complete orgasm during an erotic dream, just as normal males do. In our patient, however, the orgasm will not be accompanied by an erect penis and there will be no ejaculation. The experience is really *all in his mind,* and does not require the participation of the sex organs.

Why Can't I Feel Good All the Time?

Why is it, you must be asking now, that these pleasure centers in the brain don't keep us in a constant state of ecstasy? If the brain is so well organized to experience pleasure, why don't we experience more of it? A pessimist might even go so far as to point out that most of us will spend much more of our time being unhappy, or at least neutral, about things than we will spend in a state of unbridled joy. Or, to put it another way, why should so many people have to take drugs to experience the heights of pleasure? Why can't we just "switch on" our pleasure centers whenever we want to? The answer is that, while the brain allows us to experience intense pleasure, it is not organized so that we can do so all of the time. In fact, under normal circumstances, the brain is downright stingy about doling out intense pleasure. There are limitations to the kinds of activities that the brain can interpret as pleasurable or rewarding.

There are two closely related reasons for this state of affairs. In the first place, not all parts of the brain are equally active at all times. You can easily see this for yourself. Close your eyes for a few minutes. What happens? You don't see anything! But hold on! There's an important principle at work here. When you close your eyes, you've removed the stimulation from the nerve cells *in the brain* that are responsible for providing you with the experience of sight. By turning off the stimulation from the world around you, you have silenced the nerves that carry visual signals from the retina of your eye to the visual cortex of your brain. In so doing, you have reduced the activity of the nerve cells in the visual center of the brain. These cells normally must be active for you to have the experience of sight.

The important principle here is that the functions that are associated with specific brain centers occur only when the cells that make up those centers are *active.* The principle is quite general. It is just as true for pleasure or reward centers as it is for visual centers. Intense pleasure is experienced only when the cells in these pleasure centers are very active.

The cells in the brain that are involved in this activity-experience relationship are nerve cells, or *neurons*. These neurons are the signaling or information-processing cells of the nervous system. They differ from most of the other cells of the body in that their level of activity is not constant. They vary from second to second and from minute to minute in their excitability and in the level of their activity. It is this difference in activity level that enables them to carry out all of the complex processes that we associate with the human brain. Thinking, feeling, speaking, suffering, loving, hating, remembering—all of these are made possible by this ability of neurons to vary their level of activity. Scientists have known this for a long time, and in recent years have developed an impressive array of techniques to monitor these changes in activity level of brain cells. Some of these techniques, like PET scans that monitor energy expenditure by cells, have moved out of the laboratory and become useful diagnostic tools in medicine.

The neurons that make up the reward centers are no exception to this rule. They are not equally active at all times. Increases in their activity level are necessary for events to be rewarding. It is when these centers are most active that the experience of pleasure is most intense. The capacity to experience pleasure depends on the *activity* of the neurons in these parts of the brain. More specifically, when cells in certain portions of the brain are highly active they give rise to the subjective experience of pleasure. The more active these cells are, the more intense the pleasure.

And that points to the second reason why people are not always in a state of heightened pleasure. It has to do with the kinds of things that can make these pleasure centers highly active. In Olds's original experiments the cells were made active by the electrical stimulation supplied by the scientist. In the real world outside the laboratory, things are not so simple. Cells in the pleasure centers are not activated directly by a stimulus from the outside world; they are activated by other cells in the brain. These cells, in turn, are activated by other brain cells, which are activated by still other brain cells, and so on. Finally, at some point in this chain, neurons are found that are stimulated by input from the external world.

All this is to say that the brain's pleasure centers are isolated from various environmental inputs by neuron networks of varying complexity. These centers are located in such a way that not all interactions with the environment are equally capable of activating them.

Some behaviors, like eating, are connected to the brain's pleasure centers more directly than are other behaviors, such as learning to conjugate French verbs. Not surprisingly, most people find more pleasure in the former than in the latter. Sexual behavior leads to activity in neural pathways which are even more directly connected to pleasure centers in the brain. Accordingly, sex provides greater intensity of pleasure than does eating.

Other things, like solving arithmetic problems, are not so closely connected with the brain's reward centers. These activities are not noteworthy for producing pleasure. In some people, however, activities like these may, in fact, acquire the ability to activate reward centers. In these cases, presumably, additional neural pathways to these centers have developed in the course of living and learning. Scientists still have no idea how this happens. One thing is certain, however. This kind of acquired ability to activate pleasure centers never does so as efficiently and intensely as the inborn nerve circuits do. When was the last time that you heard anyone say that calculus was more fun than sex?

Why should the brain be constructed in this way? If pleasure is possible, why is the brain put together so that most of our actions don't bring us great pleasure? Why is it that many, if not most, actions that are engaged in repeatedly do not bring us great pleasure, at least not with any immediacy. Of course, there *are* some rewards or pleasures that poke their heads up now and then. Paydays come, even if only weekly or monthly. But life still consists of a lot of grit and grind. Thoreau seems to have had this in mind when he lamented, "Most men lead lives of quiet desperation." If he had had the knowledge that scientists have today, he might have asked, "What is it in man's brain that will permit him, or perhaps even encourage him, to engage in long, nonrewarding sequences of behavior, many of which are onerous to him? Why is the brain not organized to provide more ready access to its own centers of pleasure?"

Some insight into this question can be gained by asking what it would be like if the brain's pleasure centers *could* be activated more easily, perhaps at will. That's easy to answer. Fun and games all the time. No downside. Stock market take a tumble? Discouraged about it? No problem. Just switch on pleasure. Watch your troubles evaporate. Your kids aren't doing well in school? Your spouse is leaving you? Don't like your job? The boss hates you? Hit the pleasure switch. Why put up with feelings and emotional states that are unpleasant? Just fire up the pleasure centers for a while and chase the blues away.

Not a bad existence, at least at first glance. But there is another side to it. When you can switch on the pleasure so easily, it is easy to forget about the stock market. You can forget about your kid's lack of progress in school. You can forget about trying to salvage your marriage. And the job? Why worry about that when you're feeling so fine? An ever-present, easily available access to the heights of pleasure may divert people from tasks that are essential to their well-being, or to the well-being of those who are dependent on them. It may even divert their attention from the well-being, even the survival, of generations yet unborn. Some inkling of that possibility can be seen in Helen and Charley. They virtually gave up sex when they found the key that turned on an even more seductive pleasure.

Their key was cocaine.

Cocaine is not like arithmetic. While some people may learn to derive pleasure from solving arithmetic problems, *everyone* can derive intense pleasure from taking cocaine. Nothing special is required to hook up the drug with the brain's pleasure centers. It makes the connection naturally, like eating, like sex—only better.

What is it about the organization of the brain that accounts for this difference? Why is it that people are able to reap such immediate pleasure from taking cocaine when they are unable to do so from most other actions in which they engage?

The Evolution Connection

The human brain is the remarkable product of millions of years of evolution. Over these years the brain has developed into its current form by a process of modification of and selection from earlier forms. The modifications of these earlier forms that have "stuck," so to speak, are those which have favored the survival of the individual and the species. Many of these earlier forms can be seen today in other members of the animal kingdom. The human brain is the current model of an organ that has served its possessors well over many millennia. It provides us with capacities that far outstrip those of any of our animal relatives. Indeed, our capacities and abilities are so superior to other animal species that we have come to dominate them completely in the competition for the world's resources. In the current scheme of things, man really is the master of all that he surveys.

But the recognition of these vastly superior capabilities should not obscure the relationship between the brain of man and, say, the brain of a chimpanzee or even of a rat. Evolution is really a process of selection, modification and change. It is a conservative process which does not often favor radical innovation. It builds upon the foundations available at a given time. The changes that occur are usually, quantitatively speaking, small. The resultant qualitative changes, however, are sometimes enormous and of profound significance.

Comparing the human brain to the brains of lower animals shows clearly how distinctly human capacities emerged from a process of modification and selection. Human beings are capable of vastly greater intellectual feats than are other animals. The primary reason is that, in humans, the part of the brain known as the cerebral cortex has developed much more complexity than it has in lower animals. Most of the intellectual capabilities that are regarded as uniquely human, capabilities such as speech, are the result of this development. But virtually all of the brain structures that are found in lower animals have been preserved in man. The impressive development of human intellectual capacity has not occurred as a result of discarding brain structures that have served animals well over many millennia. On the contrary, it has occurred as an overlay to those structures. Structures and functions that have proven their worth are conserved and are common to much of the animal world.

For the most part, what has been preserved over the course of evolution are those structures and functions that are basic to the life process. Those aspects of brain organization that have furthered evolutionary success in the animal kingdom have been retained over a considerable range of species. There is much in common between the brain of man and the brain of the chimpanzee and of the other higher apes. But there is even a lot in common between the brain of man and that of the lowly rat. And, as comparisons are made with animals lower in the mammalian hierarchy, the similarities that are found lie in those structures and functions that serve to maintain life.

Breathing, eating, digestion, reproduction and other basic life processes are regulated by the brain in much the same way in humans and in lower animals.

Scientists have recently made great strides in understanding the mechanisms through which drugs like cocaine exert their influence on the brain. Many of these advances have been possible because the human brain has so much in common with the brains of other animals. It has been possible, therefore, to investigate the actions of cocaine in experimental animals with some degree of assurance that the findings would be applicable to human beings.

The picture that emerges from these investigations indicates that the human response to cocaine is not unique. It is exhibited by many other animals. Rats, for example, will administer cocaine to themselves much as people do. They will do this without being coerced. Moreover, it has become increasingly evident that the basis of the rat's eagerness to consume cocaine is probably identical to the basis of cocaine addiction in humans. That is, cocaine is attractive to humans because it acts on brain structures that are located in areas of the brain that we have in common with lower animals. Cocaine is able to exert such a powerful hold on people because it taps into brain mechanisms that are basic and fundamental to animal life.

What are the mechanisms? Simply put, pleasure. Pleasure is the powerful shaper of behavior in animals and in man. People and animals tend to do those things that bring pleasure. They try to avoid doing those things that result in pain. This basic role of pleasure and pain in guiding behavior found its most succinct expression some seventy years ago in a statement of the American psychologist, E. L. Thorndike. "Pleasure," he said, "stamps in. Pain stamps out." Parents knew about this "stamping" process long before Thorndike, of course. The judicious meting out of rewards and punishments, of pleasures and pains, is the timeless process that parents have used to insure that their children's behavior conforms to the patterns demanded by society. The larger social group, too, has always used similar means to shape conformity among its members. In this latter case, the pains or punishments and the behaviors which they are designed to stamp out have been codified in formal laws, so that all members of the social group may be aware of them.

Of even more basic interest is the biological as well as social wisdom in the uses of pleasure. If a species is to survive, it must reproduce more of its own kind. The individual members of the species must engage in those activities that promote survival. They must obtain enough food to sustain them. They must engage in mate selection and sexual behavior in order to reproduce. Finally, they must provide for the protection of their offspring until these new members of the species are able to provide for themselves.

To a large extent animals are biologically organized so that they are very likely to engage in behaviors that promote survival. The organization lies in the way that the brain is structured. The organizational plan is simple. Biological activities that have great survival value are closely connected by the nervous system to the centers of pleasure in the brain. Those activities that are essential to the survival of the individual or the species stimulate these centers and bring pleasure to the organism. The pleasure centers of the brain thus shape his behavior and increase the possibility that he will engage in the behavior again and again. Sexual behavior is the most obvious example of this kind of shaping. But the important role of the brain's pleasure centers is not limited to sex. Accumulating laboratory data have made it increasingly evident that other essential activities are influenced by these pleasure centers. Activities such as eating, and even caring for the young, are rendered more likely because of their ability to stimulate the pleasure centers of the brain.

And what is the place of cocaine in all of this? Cocaine is such a powerful and addicting drug because it is capable of directly activating reward centers in the brain. It does this chemically, and it requires no learning on the user's part. Cocaine, within seconds or minutes of its introduction into the body, activates these centers and causes the euphoria that the drug user finds so hard to resist. Cocaine rivals and may even surpass direct electrical stimulation in its ability to activate the pleasure centers. It is because of this activation that cocaine is able to exert such powerful control over the cocaine-dependent person. The individual using cocaine has found a direct route into those centers of the brain that exert profound effects in molding behavior. These centers are millions of years old and are shared with large segments of the animal kingdom. They are the very centers which, when active, play a major role in channeling the behavior of the individual into activities that are beneficial to his survival and to the survival of his species.

Unfortunately, cocaine subverts this process. It does this by divorcing the activity of the pleasure centers from other brain mechanisms. Among these other mechanisms are those that constrain the influence that the pleasure centers exert upon behavior. It is easy to see that such constraints must exist. After all, animals do not eat incessantly, even though food intake is associated with pleasure. There are many complicated factors that regulate food intake. Among these are brain mechanisms that exert regulatory control of the reward centers. The reward centers can play their important role of shaping biologically useful behavior, but the centers are themselves regulated by other brain mechanisms called forth by those behaviors. While these processes are not completely understood, it is clear that the disruption of these regulatory mechanisms upsets the balance. For example, chemical blockage of areas of the brain's hypothalamus that provide information to the reward centers reduces or eliminates the reward value of food in rats.

Cocaine perverts the behavioral shaping function of the pleasure centers. It removes the centers from their proper role in guiding behavior into highly regulated, biologically meaningful channels. It does this because it can activate the pleasure centers directly while bypassing built-in constraints upon those centers. Rather than shaping activities along biologically useful lines, the powerful influences of reward are employed only to encourage the individual to take more of the drug. Cocaine sings a siren song to the pleasure centers and enlists their powerful aid in shaping and maintaining the biologically useless activity of taking drugs.

But why is cocaine able to do this? Most drugs, after all, cannot. Is there something special about cocaine that makes it possible for it to dominate the brain in this way? The answer is that, yes, there is something special about cocaine. Cocaine affects certain nerve cells in ways that most other drugs are unable to do. To understand how cocaine does this, it is necessary to take a closer look at how these brain cells, these neurons, work. The next chapter explores the way in which cocaine exploits this process and increases the activity of neurons in the brain's reward centers.

Chapter 6

Unlocking the Pleasure Centers: How the Key Works

The nerve cells of the brain are able to vary their activity level or their state of excitation. Your ability to think, to plan, to see, to touch, to experience pain or to experience emotion is a consequence of this variation in the activity level of your neurons.

As you move along with your life, minute by minute, day by day, the ever-changing landscape of your activities and interests is reflected in, and is governed by, these constantly changing levels of activity in the neurons in your brain. These changes in activity level are, in turn, organized into changing patterns of relationships among groups of nerve cells in various parts of the brain. As you read this page, neurons in your visual pathways, beginning in the retina of your eye and traveling to the visual centers of the brain, are among the most active of all your nerve cells. If your attention is diverted by a sound, cells in the nerve circuits responsible for hearing increase their activity level and the pattern of relationships among your brain cells changes markedly. If your attention falters and your eyes slip from the page as you drift into reverie, still other neurons change their level of excitation, and other patterns of brain activity result. And so it goes, never ceasing, not even in sleep.

Saying this, however, does not really illuminate the basic task performed by the nervous system as these complex changes occur.

What these ever-varying levels of activity accomplish is the exchange of information, the basic commodity of the nervous system. As information flows from one part of the nervous system to another, in constantly shifting patterns of communication, changes in the activity of nerve cells initiate and guide this flow.

As Figure 6.1 shows, some of this information flow conveys intelligence about the outside world—how it looks, how it smells, how it sounds or tastes or feels. This information flow is made possible because some of the neurons in the nervous system are specialized to decode information about the external world. These neurons are called *receptors,* and they make up the first-line interface between the individual and his world.

It may at first seem strange to talk about "decoding" the environment. What is it about the world that is so unintelligible that it would require decoding? After all, the experience of most people would lead them to describe the world as a fairly regular, meaningful place. And yet meaning is not inherent in the world. Meaning is imposed upon it by the operations of the nervous system. William James, the American philosopher and psychologist of the late nineteenth and early twentieth centuries, characterized the world of the infant as being one big, "booming, buzzing confusion." Pressed upon from all sides by the external environment, the infant is unable to make much sense of it. Sounds and lights are not yet associated with discrete objects or events. Other people, in the beginning of extrauterine existence, are not experienced as beings clearly distinct from oneself. The vast and constantly changing panoply of the exter-

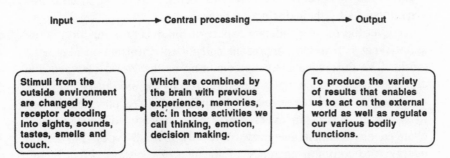

Input ──────────► Central processing ──────────► Output

| Stimuli from the outside environment are changed by receptor decoding into sights, sounds, tastes, smells and touch. | Which are combined by the brain with previous experience, memories, etc. in those activities we call thinking, emotion, decision making. | To produce the variety of results that enables us to act on the external world as well as regulate our various bodily functions. |

Fig. 6.1 Simplified diagram of information flow through the nervous system, from sensory input to processing by the brain, leading to outputs which regulate body functions and produce effects on the environment

nal world has not yet been endowed with unities of organization. Only as the child grows older and matures does the world take on more orderly dimensions, and then only because his developing nervous system is increasingly able to impose regularity on this welter of events.

The first step in this imposition of order and meaning is carried out by those specialized neurons called receptors. Receptors sort the world into meaningful categories of experience. Some of the receptors are specialized to sort the world into collections of sounds. Others sort external stimuli into collections of visual images. A different set of receptors convey information about physical objects that come into direct contact with the body. Still others sort the environment on the basis of taste or smell.

This kind of imposition of meaning on an indifferent and otherwise chaotic world goes a long way in defining the parameters of human existence. The initial sorting of the world into sensory categories operates under rigid constraints, rules of operation that are fixed for each species by evolutionary processes. While it is true that humans think differently than dogs because of the vastly superior quality of the human cerebral cortex, it is equally true that the two species experience the world differently at the receptor level. The human sensory experience of a wide range of color is undoubtedly richer than the grey-shaded world of the dog. But the dog responds to sounds that are forever out of the reach of his human master, and his olfactory world is infinitely more varied. What would human experience be like if we were able to respond to the range of odors that constitute reality for the dog? What kind of a world would it be if we were able to identify all of our friends and acquaintances by their distinctive odors?

And yet the most significant aspect of this receptor function is not simply that it provides important categorical information about the world. The difference in receptor coding of the world between dog and man is of little importance compared to the *similarity* in receptor function in the two species. What all of this receptor activity has in common is that, in every case, these specialized neurons have changed environmental energy of widely diverse types into neural energy, the common currency of the nervous system. Electromagnetic energy has been changed into vision. Pressure changes in the surrounding air have been turned into sound. Chemical molecules in the nasal cavities have been changed into smells and pressure changes on the skin have been transmuted into touch and pain. Receptor action renders the environment intelligible because it changes external information, which exists in a form that most cells in the nervous system cannot process, into neural energy, a form that can be manipulated by the brain.

This process is called *transduction*. While the receptor is specialized to respond to some particular aspect of the environment, this ability would be of no use whatsoever if the information about the environment could not be passed on to other neurons. Receptors derive their utility from the fact that they can *communicate* information about the external world to other nerve cells that are unable to process this information on their own. The ability of receptors to decode the environment would be of no use if these cells were not able also to transmit the result of their actions to other neurons.

An analogous statement can be made about the output of the system shown in Figure 6.1. The muscles that move you would be impotent if they did not receive impulses to initiate and guide them. From a toddler's first halting steps to the smoothly coordinated stride of an Olympic sprinter, from the random babblings of the newborn to the measured cadences of Macbeth, the entire range of motion and locomotion is possible only because the muscular activation is the end product of numerous and smoothly integrated impulses.

The impulses come, of course, from the nervous system. And it is the nervous system, or rather some defect in it, that is at fault in most of the pathological conditions that are referred to as disorders of movement. Parkinsonism, Huntington's disease, multiple sclerosis, all of these grave disorders that present motor disorders as their most readily recognized symptoms, all of these are the result of failed or compromised impulse transmission in the nervous system. The activation of the muscles is the end result of a complex communication chain in which messages of considerable sophistication have been passed from neuron to neuron.

Finally, thinking, feeling, imagining, wanting, loving, hating, the entire gamut of experiences that marks us as distinctly human, all of these would be impossible if one neuron could not transmit information to another.

Neurons communicate with one another. They exchange messages among themselves. And they do this with a degree of organizational complexity that makes even the most powerful of modern computers seem simple by comparison. Everything you do is dependent upon this intercommunication among brain cells. The aggregate activity of the brain is the result of ten billion neurons passing messages to one another. If individual neurons could not do this, none of the impressive operations of the human intellect would be possible.

Clinical medicine is full of examples of the disastrous consequences of the failure of this communication process. The movement disorders mentioned above are only the tip of the neurological disease iceberg. Alzheimer's disease is the result of the massive loss of the ability of certain neurons to exchange messages with other neurons. Furthermore, it now seems likely that mental disorders that have defied understanding for centuries, disorders like schizophrenia, depression, compulsions and anxiety states, are also the result of compromised communication among specific neurons.

Appreciation of this fact has led to the development of medications that are effective in treating these conditions. These drugs act by altering selective aspects of message transmission in the patient's brain. The key word here is *selective*. Different drugs are used to treat different disorders because drugs vary in the neurons that they affect. That is, drugs vary in the message channels in which they produce their effects. This notion of the selective action of drugs is an important determinant of cocaine's ability to produce dependence and abuse.

Stepping Into the Communications Loop

It is worth repeating: The business of neurons is communication, the interchange of information. The vast collection of nerve cells that we call the brain is the most remarkable communication center we know. To be human is precisely to be an incredibly efficient information processor.

There are, however, numerous circumstances in which it is possible to modify this process of message transmission to our great advantage. In some such circumstances it is possible to *interfere* with the information processing or communicating ability of some neurons while leaving other neurons unaffected. Some very useful drugs do this. General anesthetics, for example, when administered correctly, render some portions of the brain incapable of receiving and transmitting information from other parts of the brain or from cells in other parts of the body. The neurons in these areas, neurons whose activity is essential to a conscious appreciation of what is happening to us, are taken out of the communication loop. Anesthetic drugs can therefore be administered to bring about the blessed state of unconsciousness that makes surgery possible.

Note, however, that one of the characteristics that makes general anesthetics useful drugs is that, if administered correctly, they leave intact the ability of some neurons to engage in information processing and communication. The unaffected neurons continue their business as if nothing had happened. Among the neurons that are left unscathed are the nerve cells and circuits that keep you breathing while you are anesthetized.

Consider another example of altered message transmission. Consider for a moment those drugs that are derived from the opium poppy. These drugs are called opiate narcotics. No other drug is capable of relieving pain to the same degree, and with the same selectivity, as are the opiate narcotics. Other drugs, like the general anesthetics, are capable of making you oblivious to pain, but they lack the selectivity of the opiates. Even alcohol can relieve pain if administered in sufficient quantity. But in the case of general anesthetics or alcohol the pain is relieved only by rendering the patient unconscious. The great advantage of the opiate narcotics is that they compromise the communication ability of those nerve cells that convey information about pain while leaving other neurons able to communicate as usual. Halstead led a long productive life while addicted to morphine. He, like patients taking narcotics, was still able to see, hear, smell, taste and think coherently. The narcotics enable patients to be up and about and carry on with their lives.

The opiates illustrate a general principle of considerable importance. Many drugs act on specific neurons in specific areas of the nervous system, while leaving other neurons in other portions of the nervous system largely unaffected. This is why different drugs are used to treat different malfunctions of the nervous system. Opiates are not used to treat schizophrenics. Drugs that are used to treat schizophrenics are not used as pain relievers. General anesthetics are not used to bring about sedation, a milder form of depression of the central nervous system. Valium, which *is* used to bring about sedation, would not be used to depress the CNS in order to perform an appendectomy.

This specificity of drug action exists because there is a relationship between the chemical structure of the drug and the chemical composition of the cells on which the drug acts. The structure of a drug determines where and how it will exert its action in the body. The site and mechanism of action of the drug, in other words, is determined by its chemical architecture. Drugs work only on those parts of the nervous system where the "chemistry is right." This aspect of drug action has profound consequences for drug abuse and the way in which we elect to approach the problems that drug abuse poses for our society.

Before pursuing these consequences, however, we must follow in more detail the possibilities inherent in the idea of using drugs to alter communication in the nervous system. In the examples already considered, the information processing or communicating ability of the neurons was adversely affected by the drug. Opiates interfere with the ability of some neurons to communicate with other neurons. Anesthetics compromise the communicating ability of still other neurons. But there is no logical reason to suspect that all drugs must exert this kind of negative action on nerve cells. Other drugs might have quite the opposite kind of effects on their target neurons. Such drugs would, in some sense, enhance the ability of these neurons to engage in communication and information processing. In these cases, drugs would increase the amount of information flow from one neuron to another.

A case in point is the drug L-dopa, used to alleviate the symptoms of parkinsonism. This disease is the result of the deterioration of the brain's nigrostriatal pathway. These neurons connect a portion of the brain called the substantia nigra to another portion called the caudate nucleus. As the neurons of the nigrostriatal pathway deteriorate, message transmission in this information circuit is impaired. The result is the appearance of the tremors and poorly coordinated movement that are characteristic of parkinsonism. The drug L-dopa restores some of the lost message-transmitting ability to these neurons. The result is an amelioration of the clinical signs of the disorder.

But increased message transmission is not always an unalloyed blessing. Its results are not always therapeutic. Some drugs can facilitate message transmission to the point that the channels are overstimulated. In this case, brain function, rather than being improved by the drug, is liable to become pathological. Information transfer from one neuron to another is garbled, and the precision of message transmission is impaired.

Cocaine is just such a drug.

Cocaine, like opiates, alters the communicating ability of the neurons that it affects. Unlike the opiates, however, cocaine affects *its* target neurons by *increasing* the amount of their information-passing activity. And, unlike L-dopa, cocaine acts primarily on neurons that are functioning normally. Rather than nudging underperforming neurons in the direction of normal output, cocaine pushes normally functioning neurons into a heightened level of activity which can impair the normal operation of the brain.

But how does cocaine do this? Is there a relationship between this action of cocaine and its ability to produce the kind of pleasure that people will seek out over and over again? It will be easier to answer these questions following a more detailed look at the basic mechanism of *normal* message transmission in the brain.

If It's Chemical We Must Be Communicating

A close look at two neurons that communicate with one another reveals that there is a physical gap between the neuron that is transmitting the message and the neuron that receives it. This anatomical relationship is shown in Figure 6.2.

The close association of the two neurons across this gap is called a *synapse.* The neuron on the "upstream," or message-originating side of the synapse, is called the *presynaptic* neuron. The neuron of the "downstream," or message-receiving side of the synapse, is called the *postsynaptic* neuron. The process of message transmission across this synaptic gap, or *synaptic cleft,* is called synaptic transmission.

Consider the problem of message transmission from the standpoint of the nerve cells involved. Suppose that you were a presynaptic neuron that had just come into possession of some exciting new information. Naturally, you would be just itching to pass on the news to your neighbors, other neurons. This means that you would have to find some way to get the information across the synaptic cleft that separates you from them. Since you have no mobility and cannot, therefore, draw closer to your neighboring neuron, you will

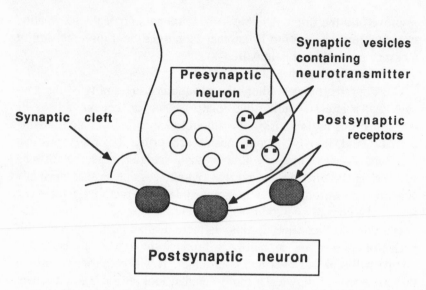

Fig. 6.2 Diagram of a simple synapse, showing presynaptic vesicles and postsynaptic receptors

have to find some way to launch a message across the gap. You must find a way to package the information so it can be sent across the cleft to the postsynaptic neuron. You must also insure that your message is packaged so that the postsynaptic neuron will be able to read it.

The way in which the problem is solved in the mammalian nervous system is to package the information in chemical form and then send these chemical messengers across the synaptic cleft. Message transmission in the human brain is chemical in nature. The chemicals which are secreted by the presynaptic neuron are called *neurotransmitters*. If message transmission in the brain is to work correctly, the presynaptic neuron must secrete the correct amount of neurotransmitter at the correct time.

The presynaptic neuron, however, could do all of this without any guarantee that communication would take place. Communication is, after all, not a solitary process. There's no sense sending forth messages, no matter how important they may be, if no one is listening. If neural communication is to occur, the postsynaptic neuron must indeed be paying attention. In the nervous system the nerve cells that receive the information are every bit as important as the neurons that deliver the message. Indeed, in the case of some drug actions the receiving neurons are even more important than are the transmitting nerve cells.

And just how does a neuron "pay attention"? By chemical means, of course. Receiving neurons will be able to "understand" the chemical messages launched in their direction if they are able to recognize the particular neurotransmitter that is knocking at their door. Communication in the nervous system proceeds because neurons are able to perform both input and output functions. They signal other neurons by the release of neurotransmitter and they respond to chemicals to which they are exposed.

The recognition function is carried out by a portion of the nerve cell that is called its *neurotransmitter receptor.* This receptor is, so to speak, a biological "lock" into which the neurotransmitter "key" fits. The analogy is a good one. As it turns out, part of the complexity of the brain lies in the fact that several different chemicals are used as neurotransmitters. If message transmission under these conditions is not to be hopelessly garbled, it is essential that there be a match between the transmitter that is released and the receptor that responds to it. This match is guaranteed by a sort of chemical fit between the transmitter and the receptor. The lock and key fit because of their chemical structures.

This type of message transmission involves enormous subtleties of organization. The process is closely regulated in the brain, and any disruption of this organization, any deviation from optimal conditions of interneuron communication, can drastically affect the brain's ability to function appropriately. It is, in fact, just such subtle derangements in the process of synaptic transmission that are thought to cause serious mental disorders like schizophrenia and depression. Pharmacological treatment of these disorders, in turn, is based on the attempt to return this process to normal.

Yes, You Can Get Too Much of a Good Thing!

The secretion of chemical messages is essential if the brain is to function. No chemical messenger secretion means no brain function. It is also the case, however, that the *amount* of neurotransmitter released must be closely regulated. Not only must the message-generating neuron, the presynaptic one, secrete the neurotransmitter, but there must also be a mechanism that guarantees that the receptor is *not overstimulated* by the communication. Not only is it possible, as in the case of anesthetics, to derange the brain by interfering with the ability of neurons to communicate, but it is also possible to derange the brain by enhancing the ability of these cells to transmit messages.

You are probably already familiar with the disastrous consequences of overstimulation of the postsynaptic neuron by abnormal amounts of neurotransmitter. The insects that you spray with common aerosol insecticides die because of this sort of chemical-induced overstimulation. It is important to realize that the stimulation is not caused directly by the poison. Rather, the poison causes overstimulation of the postsynaptic receptor by the brain's own neurotransmitter. Some of the most potent nerve toxins known to man, the kind that make up a major portion of the chemical warfare arsenal of modern states, kill their victims in exactly this way.

The task of avoiding overstimulation is carried out by neurons in two different ways. In some cases, the neurotransmitter is destroyed by enzymes before overstimulation can occur. This is what normally happens with the nerve cells on which insecticides exert their lethal action. The neurons in that case are those that make synapses with muscle fibers rather than with other neurons. The message conveyed by the neurotransmitter is, in this case, "Contract!" Receptors on the muscle fibers recognize this message, cause the muscle to contract and the result is movement or locomotion. The amount of neurotransmitter stimulating the receptor is closely regulated so that excessive muscular contraction does not occur. The regulation is carried out by an enzyme that modifies the chemical structure of the neurotransmitter. The enzyme changes the shape of the key so that it no longer fits into the lock.

How the system is changed when the insecticide is present! The toxin is absorbed into the bloodstream and delivered to the synapses where muscle contraction is being directed. The enzyme is unable to distinguish between molecules of neurotransmitter and molecules of poison, and it tries to alter the insecticide just as it does the neurotransmitter. But whereas the neurotransmitter has no effect on the enzyme that degrades it, the poison molecule "fights back." It holds the enzyme fast so that it is no longer able to inactivate the neurotransmitter. The result is that the neurotransmitter overstimulates the muscles and they remain in a state of chronic contraction. Some of the muscles affected are those that control breathing, and the insect dies of respiratory paralysis.

In the neurons that are most directly involved with cocaine, the problem of overstimulation is solved by a different means. It is solved by the presynaptic neuron itself. To insure that the postsynaptic receptor is not overstimulated by the neurotransmitter, the presynaptic neuron takes the chemical back after the message has been delivered. The process is called reuptake. The presynaptic neuron is able to secrete the correct amount of chemical messenger and recall it appropriately so that the receiving neuron is not overstimulated. Figure 6.3 gives a simplified view of these two processes of message regulation.

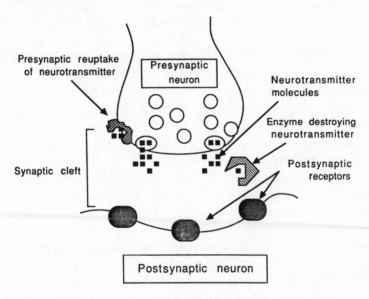

Fig. 6.3 Synaptic message termination by enzymatic destruction or presynaptic reuptake

Drug Action Is Like Real Estate: The Three Most Important Variables Are Location, Location and Location

Many drug effects are known to occur because of the actions of the chemicals on some aspects of synaptic transmission.

- L-dopa acts to increase the amount of neurotransmitter available for release by the deteriorating neurons in the nigrostriatal tract.
- Opiates act by reducing the ability of neurons carrying pain messages to transmit their information across the synapse.

- Drugs that are used to treat schizophrenia affect the synapse in at least two ways. In the short run, they modify the message-receiving capability of the post-synaptic neuron. This action, in the long run, alters the message-transmitting capacity of the presynaptic neuron.
- Drugs that are used to treat depression exert their effects by short-run effects on the presynaptic neuron. These effects, in turn, produce long-run changes in the functioning of the postsynaptic receptor.

In all of these cases it is essential to remember that many drugs are more or less selective in their actions. They act on some neurons and not others. In the case of drugs that exert important actions on the synapse, they act on some synapses more readily than they do on others.

Cocaine is no exception to this rule. The reward-related actions of cocaine do not take place everywhere in the brain. They occur only where the "chemistry is right." Moreover, these actions occur at the synapse, a fact that means that the chemistry is right at some synapses and not at others. Cocaine's enhancement of activity in the brain's pleasure circuits, in other words, occurs because of the drug's ability to modify synaptic transmission in these particular circuits and not willy-nilly throughout the brain.

Cocaine has other actions, to be sure. These other actions underlie the local anesthetic effect that has been discussed in the preceding chapters. Such actions, which are *not* exerted immediately upon the synapse, are an exception to the notion of selectivity of drug action. They will occur in any nerve, in any part of the nervous system, to which cocaine is applied. It is the more selective synaptic actions of the drug that are strongly related to the pleasure producing, abuse-potential effects of the drug.

Cocaine has such direct access to the synapses that are involved in the brain's pleasure circuitry because of its relationship to the neurotransmitters in those circuits. A number of different chemicals serve as neurotransmitters in the human brain, though scientists are not in agreement on their exact number. Some of these neurotransmitters are widely distributed throughout the brain, whereas others are localized in specific areas. Cocaine has the ability to interact with a transmitter that is heavily concentrated in the brain's pleasure circuits.

But there is more to this neurotransmitter variety. Consider the lock-and-key analogy. If the key (neurotransmitter) used by one neuron is different from the key used by another neuron, the locks (receptor) that they open are also different. A changed transmitter means a changed receptor. The change in neurotransmitter from one synapse to another implies that the chemistry of the entire synapse is changed. For drugs that act on the synapse this leads to several ideas of profound importance.

- Different communication channels in the brain may require different neurotransmitters.
- To say that the "chemistry is right" is to say that a drug may affect one neurotransmitter more than another.
- Drugs act selectively by altering communication by one transmitter and not another.
- Drugs may vary in their effects because their chemical structure allows them access to different communication channels.

The brain, in other words, has a chemical organization as well as an anatomical organization. Its various functions may be carried out by different transmitters. It becomes a meaningful question, therefore, to inquire into the chemical organization of the brain, and in particular into the ways in which specific drugs can affect this organization. Specifically, with regard to cocaine, is the perception of pleasure heavily influenced by the activity of a particular neurotransmitter? If so, what is the relationship between that transmitter and drugs that elicit strong feelings of pleasure?

The Chemistry of Pleasure

One of the best known neurotransmitters is a chemical called *dopamine*. Dopamine is not widely distributed in the brain, but is concentrated in three or four specific brain areas. About 75 percent of it, as a matter of fact, is found in the nigrostriatal tract, which is involved in parkinsonism. It is in these areas that the "chemistry is right" for the drug L-dopa. Consequently, the drug acts at the appropriate site in the brain to bring about relief from the symptoms of the disorder.

Another brain area rich in dopamine-secreting neurons is called the ventral tegmental area (VTA). Cells in the VTA stimulate another brain region called the nucleus accumbens. These structures are an important component of the pleasure centers of the brain. In fact, these dopamine-secreting neurons are one of the major inputs to the pleasure centers. These dopamine neurons are one of the most, perhaps *the* most, important source of messages that the pleasure centers receive. When these dopamine neurons are highly active, in other words, the pleasure centers of the brain are being bombarded with messages that say, in effect, "Something good is going on!"

Message termination in these particular neurons is accomplished by presynaptic reuptake. If this process were to fail or be weakened in some way, the input of messages to the pleasure centers would be increased over and above that normally conveyed by the usual release of transmitter. The brain in this case would overinterpret the extent to which it was true that "something good is going on!"

Cocaine induces these dopamine neurons to send precisely this sort of message to the pleasure centers. Here is how the process works. When cocaine is absorbed into the bloodstream, it is carried rapidly to the brain by the ample blood supply that serves that organ. Very quickly after administration, cocaine appears in large amounts in all parts of the brain. Most important, some of the drug finds it way into the vicinity of the dopamine neurons. Once there, cocaine increases the rate of message flow from these dopamine neurons to the pleasure centers. It is by this action on dopamine nerve cells that cocaine causes hyperstimulation of the pleasure centers of the brain.

Some of the mechanisms by which cocaine does this are beginning to be understood. The drug prevents dopamine neurons from monitoring and modulating their own message transmission. These neurons are able to *deliver* messages to the pleasure centers, but cocaine destroys their ability to control the *amount* of information conveyed. To put it another way, the actual input of messages to the pleasure centers is left unaffected by the drug. However, the message which is delivered is magnified out of all proportion to the amount of neurotransmitter actually released by the presynaptic neuron.

How is this accomplished? By the simple but very effective mechanism shown in Figure 6.4. Cocaine interferes with the reuptake ability of the presynaptic neuron. Because of its chemical structure, cocaine is able to prevent the dopamine neurons from taking back the neurotransmitter chemical that they release. Since this sort of reuptake by the presynaptic neuron is the way in which message transmission is terminated in these cells, the drug causes an unceasing stimulation of the cells that receive the neurotransmitter. Although the mechanism is different, the effect on synaptic transmission is very similar to the effect produced by the insecticide. Reduced neuronal reuptake means more neurotransmitter acting at the receptor over a longer time. The consequence is an unusually high degree of activation of the postsynaptic neuron, the cells which are inputs to the brain's pleasure centers.

Finally, as always, the brain interprets its own experience. Just as activity in auditory regions of the brain is interpreted as sound; just as activity in visual areas of the brain is interpreted as sight; so, too, increased activity in the pleasure centers is interpreted as "Something good is going on!"

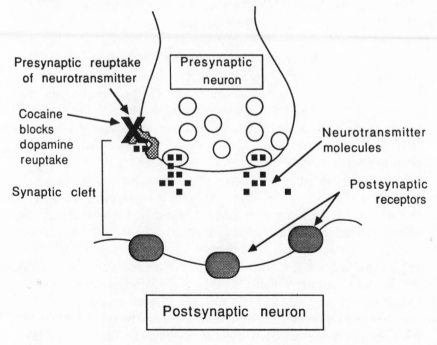

Fig. 6.4 Cocaine blockade of presynaptic reuptake of neurotransmitter

The Reuptake Story Reconsidered

So cocaine is able to block the reuptake of dopamine, and this action is an important determinant of its addiction potential. But why? What enables cocaine to do this? Why cocaine and dopamine, and why is the juxtaposition of the two so important?

The key to understanding all of this is found in the concept of a *drug receptor*. A drug receptor is a cell component having a particular three-dimensional shape. The receptor is usually (but not always) found to be a macromolecular complex on the membrane of the cell. (A macromolecular complex is a fancy name for a large molecule which can be shown to consist of a collection of smaller, recognizable molecules that work together as one. When they occur as a complex, they have unique properties.)

The receptor, in other words, is a component of the cell with which the drug can interact. A drug's effects are the direct consequence of this interaction. The principle is this: Drugs produce effects in proportion to their ability to interact with a biological receptor, that is, to fit it as a lock fits a key.

Most of the biological effects of drugs are receptor-mediated. That is, a given biological effect requires drug stimulation of the receptor as a first step. Put another way, the biological effects of different drugs vary because the drugs activate different receptors. The receptor is crucial. It is, in effect, a biological "window" on the world of certain molecular substances. If the window is not "opened" by the drug, the person remains unaware of the presence of the drug and is unaffected by it. Receptors determine the types of biological response to a drug that a person can have. The selectivity of drug effects, to the extent that it exists, is the result of a chemical match between the drug and some cellular receptor.

There are two specific aspects to this drug-receptor interaction that account for its great importance. First, a given receptor can interact effectively with only a limited class of drugs. Valium, for example, can act at Valium receptors and opiates can act at opiate receptors. They are not interchangeable. Since receptor activation is the essential first step in the biological response to drugs, Valium cannot be used to relieve pain in the same way as opiates can.

Secondly, different receptors have different biological functions because they are located on different cell types. The subtlety here lies in the fact that brain cells differ enormously among themselves.

Among the important variations is that they differ significantly in the type of receptor that they possess. Not all neurons possess Valium receptors. Not all brain cells possess opiate receptors, and so on. Neurons differ, therefore, in the type of drug to which they can respond.

Cocaine and dopamine are related in the chain of events that leads from drug-taking to addiction because the presynaptic dopamine neuron is, in a sense, "ready" for cocaine. In other words, there are cocaine receptors on these neurons. Cocaine can therefore enter into a lock-and-key relationship with the receptors on these cells. This drug-receptor interaction initiates a response from the cell, one component of which is the impairment of the cell's ability to engage in the reuptake of its own transmitter. While the entire story is by no means known to scientists, this action of cocaine appears to be crucial to the drug's ability to produce the strong craving experienced by the cocaine user. In Chapter 9 I will point out how this relationship between a drug and its receptor might be exploited to develop drugs that are even more addicting then cocaine.

James Olds unearthed areas in the brain that have come to be called pleasure centers or reward centers. He found that animals would stimulate themselves repeatedly in these areas, ignoring other aspects of their environment as they concentrated on obtaining self-stimulation. Scientists now know what Olds could not then have known. Namely, that stimulation of these areas was rewarding because it caused dopamine to be released in supernormal amounts, and this release of dopamine led to activation of these primitive portions of the brain. Rewarding brain stimulation monopolizes the interest of the animal to such a degree because it activates areas of the brain that have directed survival functions throughout evolutionary history. The reward centers convey the message "What you're doing now is important and good. Keep it up!"

Cocaine, acting through these dopamine neurons, produces the same kinds of events in the brain. And it does it even more directly than does electrical stimulation of the classic pleasure centers. Immediately after being absorbed into the bloodstream, cocaine is delivered to the brain. It quickly reaches those areas deep within the brain where dopamine neurons are found. At these sites cocaine prolongs the action of the neurotransmitter and leads to hyperstimulation by dopamine of the postsynaptic neurons. The result is immediate and overpowering stimulation of the same brain pathways that are activated by stimulation of Olds's pleasure centers. The brain structures activated are phylogenetically old and contain mechanisms that have evolved because they have contributed to survival. Cocaine use, in other words, leads to primitive pleasure that the organism is biologically programmed to appreciate. No learning required. No experience necessary.

Cheer Up! The Worst Is Yet to Come!

So cocaine acts at cocaine receptors to produce the synaptic effects that can so easily result in abuse and addiction. Unfortunately, the story does not end there. The drug-receptor relationship is even more subtle than this. In addition to being capable of distinguishing between drugs that do and do not fit, receptors are able to distinguish among drugs that *do* fit. What this means is that the neuron can produce different responses to two different drugs, both of which fit its receptor very well. Some drugs that fit the receptor will lead to its activation, thereby initiating a biological response of the neuron to this drug. Another drug which fits the receptor equally well, and in some cases even better, will not lead to activation of the receptor. The expected biological response will not occur.

The delicacy of this drug-receptor relationship can be seen in the actions of two drugs that act at the opiate receptor—morphine and Naloxone. Both drugs fit the opiate receptor very well. Their architecture is appropriate to the site. Yet they have different actions on the receptor. Morphine activates the receptor and produces pain relief. Naloxone, although it binds to the receptor as well as morphine (in fact even better), fails to activate it and does not produce analgesia. Naloxone binds to the opiate receptor so well, in fact, that if both drugs are present in the system, Naloxone will move morphine off of the receptor and prevent it from producing its effects.

Because the opiate receptor distinguishes between these two drugs, Naloxone can produce spectacular effects. If it is administered to a morphine or heroin addict, it will quickly displace these drugs from the opiate receptors, and the activation of these receptors ceases. That is the equivalent of a sudden removal of the other drugs from the system. Abruptly, a withdrawal syndrome appears. The individual has gone cold turkey.

Drug receptors are exceedingly important biological entities. The more that is known about them the more it becomes possible to tailor-make drugs to achieve specific results. For example, the accumulating knowledge of the opiate receptor (actually there are several subtypes of these, just to complicate things!) may lead to the development of pain relievers that are as potent as morphine but lack morphine's addiction potential.

There are several aspects to all of this receptor business that are relevant to the cocaine problem.

1. In actuality, there are several different dopamine receptors. Scientists are not in agreement on their exact number. What is apparent at the present time is that the different receptors, whatever their number, differ in some important ways. In response to dopamine they initiate or mediate a variety of communication processes in the brain. It is not yet known which of these processes is most involved in the effects of cocaine on dopamine neurons. (Keep in mind here, that the addictive properties of cocaine are, in a sense, indirect results of its action at the dopamine synapse. Cocaine blockade of reuptake exaggerates the *normal* response of the receptor to dopamine.)

2. In spite of all that is known about cocaine, the exact nature of the cocaine receptor has not yet been determined, although scientists do have suggestions, hypotheses and hunches. There is even some evidence that there are several different types of cocaine receptors.

3. As scientists piece together more details about the way in which cocaine interacts with biological receptors, and the way in which these interactions activate the brain's pleasure circuitry, it is highly likely that they will develop drugs with even greater and more selective action on these centers. Such drugs would have a potential for abuse and addiction that would make cocaine look mild by comparison.

Chapter 7

How Bad Is It? The Scope of the Cocaine Problem

Toting up some numbers is the conventional way to figure out how bad the cocaine problem is. Numbers like the following:

- There are an estimated five to six million regular users of cocaine in the United States.
- Data compiled in 1988 indicate that there are about 21 million people in this country who have tried the drug at least once.
- The same data indicate that about 2.5 million people have tried crack at least once.
- Drug-abuse deaths involving cocaine in the United States doubled from the last half of 1986 to the first half of 1989.
- In 1988, one-half million children from twelve to seventeen years of age had used cocaine during the past year. In young adults from eighteen to twenty-five years of age, 3.5 million had used cocaine in the past year.
- In 1988, 245 out of 1,099 bills introduced in the United

States House of Representatives were drug-related. Fully one-fifth of newly contemplated legislation was concerned with drugs. When the time necessary to see these bills through the normal legislative process is considered, one-fifth may be a serious underestimate of the legislative time and effort that is devoted to the drug problem.

- In 1989, Federal agencies seized 181,363 pounds of cocaine. This is almost fifteen times as much cocaine as was seized in a comparable time period in 1982.

What do such numbers tell you? Obviously they mean that a lot of people are using cocaine. But numbers alone don't tell the story. In fact, in unvarnished form they may even obscure the problem. Some way must be found to associate meaning with the statistics. The data must be interpreted.

The usual way of finding meaning in statistics that purport to describe a social problem is to associate the numbers with some estimates of *cost*. Society generally considers an activity to be a problem when the cost of that activity to the social group becomes unacceptable. Drunk driving constitutes a problem because its costs include traffic fatalities, disabling injuries, rising insurance rates and the loss to society of young lives prematurely snuffed out. More generally, alcoholism is regarded as a problem because of an even wider array of costs. These include lost work-place productivity, the expense of treatment and rehabilitative efforts, domestic violence, child abuse, family disintegration, and so forth.

An analysis of costs in this fashion usually makes explicit the *benefits* that would accrue to society if the problem could be solved. Any program which is proposed to alleviate the problem can then be evaluated in terms of this anticipated benefit. That is, the program in question will itself cost something, and this cost can be weighed against the benefits that are expected from it if it is successful in alleviating the problem. That is to say, the desirability of a program can be measured by performing a *cost-benefit analysis*.

In some areas of public health, the formulation of a problem in these terms is rather straightforward. Consider the question of AIDS. The dimensions of an AIDS epidemic can be estimated by conventional techniques. The first order of business is to assess the current state of affairs. Epidemiologists have developed an impressive array of survey and demographic methods designed to accomplish this. Areas of major concentrations of the disease are identified and characterized in terms of pertinent demographic variables. This analysis yields useful information concerning the most important concentrations of HIV, the presumed causative virus. The transmission of the disease is studied so that the major avenues by which the virus spreads can be identified. Then, under various assumptions about conditions likely to obtain in the near future, sophisticated statistical methods can be used to predict the spread of infection and the outbreak of disease.

Given these kinds of data it is possible to associate costs with the disease, in terms analogous to those used in discussing alcoholism. Furthermore, the predictions based upon these data allow one to anticipate the cost of the disease to society in the near future and in the long term. How many hospital beds will be required in the year 2000? What will be the cost of treatment for AIDS patients over the next ten years? Will these costs overburden the health care system? Will it be possible to keep health insurance premiums at or near their present levels? Or will the costs of the disease be so large that premiums will have to grow beyond the ability of any but the wealthy to pay? Will insurance companies simply "opt out" of the AIDS business, leaving large numbers of sick people with no resources of their own, leaving them to the mercy of a government that may or may not be disposed to help them?

Associating costs with the disease in this fashion permits a comparison with the costs of programs which are proposed to reduce or eliminate the disease.

All of this is pretty standard fare in public health circles. Basically the procedure is:

1. Ascertain the present magnitude of the problem.
2. Discover the means by which the problem grows and spreads.
3. Predict the likely size of the problem at a given time in the future.
4. Estimate the resources that will be required to deal with a problem of the size projected.
5. Predict the cost of providing these resources in the future.

6. In the interim, devise programs designed to reduce the projected size of the problem and the costs associated with it.

Analyses like these can be made in the case of cocaine. As in the case of drunk driving and alcohol addiction, social costs can be associated with cocaine use. The costs are huge, as might be expected. They fall into many of the same categories that are usually associated with alcohol addiction, or with drug abuse in general. But in the case of cocaine, and the future beyond cocaine, this approach to assessing costs is inadequate.

The problem of costs associated with cocaine use is more involved than this type of analysis suggests. On the one hand, there are costs associated with the rampant use of cocaine that are usually ignored by many of the authorities that preach solutions to the problem. In some instances, these costs are simply not appreciated by the people formulating the programs. In other cases, these costs are ignored because they would draw too much attention to how bad the problem really is. The people responsible for drawing up programs to alleviate the cocaine problem are usually the same individuals who have formulated programs in the past. To say that the problem is worse now than it was at an earlier time is to admit that earlier programs have not been outstanding successes.

Making these kinds of costs explicit would focus attention on the important benefits that would result if cocaine use were brought under control. If the benefits yet to be reaped are highly desirable, as these certainly are, people are likely to be more demanding that *new* solutions be tried and that *new* people be brought in to implement them. None of this increased public awareness is apt to be sought by those currently in a position to formulate policy.

I will refer to these not-so-willingly-discussed costs of cocaine abuse as the *hidden costs* of the problem.

Furthermore, there are a number of poorly appreciated costs associated with several of the proposed programs for "cleaning up the mess." Discussion of these costs is usually avoided, either because they are not understood by the proponents of these programs or because they raise embarrassing questions about their long-run political effects. These costs could be referred to as the *price-of-success costs*. It is exceedingly important to understand the nature of both of these price tags because, in the end, it is the American citizen who bears the burden.

The hidden costs of the cocaine epidemic are difficult or impossible to state in quantitative terms. Nevertheless, in the long run they are more destructive to social order than are the more easily categorized costs that usually receive most attention. Costs in this category, if endured long enough, tear at the very fabric of a free society. They include:

1.   *The cost to innocent victims of crimes.*

No one knows exactly what proportion of day-to-day crime is committed by people solely to obtain money to buy drugs, but most knowledgeable people suspect that the percentage is quite large.

Many of these costs are not easily measured in dollars and cents.

• The psychological and emotional torment of the victims are agonizingly real. Hospital and doctor bills are an inadequate representation of their pain.

• The fear and apprehension of the victim of an armed assault may well be more costly than his actual financial loss. He now lives in a much more hostile world. Strangers are regarded with suspicion. Certain streets, perhaps whole areas of town, are now avoided. The victim's life has been drastically altered.

• The feeling of having been violated, of no longer being safe in one's home, a feeling that is common to the burglary victim, may persist long after stolen objects have been replaced. In some ways, this may be the worst of all. Streets, neighborhoods, areas can be avoided. You can't avoid your house, however, without its ceasing to be your home.

Costs such as these are measured in fear and uncertainty and a loss in individual freedom. There is a growing consensus that the world is no longer a safe place. People tend increasingly to cower behind locked and bolted doors.

All of these results of the cocaine epidemic add up to an intolerable burden. The collective loss of freedom of movement suffered by the people of a society terrified by out-of-control street crime represents one of the major costs of the cocaine disaster.

2. *The cost to public confidence in "the system."*

Hardly a week goes by when we do not read accounts of how cocaine money has corrupted police, bankers, judges, lawyers and other public officials. One of the reasons voiced by some military authorities for not wanting to involve their troops in the domestic "war on cocaine" was their fear that the soldier at the interface between illicit drugs and society was very likely to be corrupted by the opportunity to turn an easy buck. There are enormous sums of "easy money" to be made in the cocaine trade or in the activities that it spawns. When this money is used to bribe, influence or undermine the basic institutions of society, cynicism is bred among the body politic. "Everybody's doing it," "Who can you trust?" "Take what you can get," and similar sentiments become increasingly common. People lose confidence in the very institutions that undergird a feeling of solidarity and a sense of community. Cocaine money has the potential to destroy our belief in the workability of the system.

3. *The cost of dehumanizing a society that becomes increasingly inured to violence.*

What is important here is not just the violence that one may experience directly. It is the violence that has become the normal background to life in the United States. It is street violence that has attained the status of permanent warfare among rival cocaine gangs and between gangs and law enforcement personnel. The constant barrage of killings, and the ever-increasing level of firepower used, make it more likely that many of us will live in true urban battlefields.

The arms race associated with this battle is equally frightening. Many commentators have looked with alarm at this escalation of violence. There is, however, a neglected aspect to this urban warfare that affects our society in subtle, insidious, and largely unnoticed ways. Our police departments, for example, in order to oppose the firepower of the gangs employ ever more powerful and sophisticated armaments. SWAT teams, with their characteristic clothing, assault rifles and other gear reminiscent of a Special Forces brigade, increasingly assume the character of paramilitary groups. Indeed, some law enforcement units now receive a part of their training from special forces in the military.

One result of this course of events is the creation in many local police departments of a feeling of isolation from the citizens they are sworn to protect. This is not difficult to understand .if the streets become more dangerous every day, and everyone is perceived to be a potential enemy. The fact remains, however, that to the extent that our police officers regard everyone as a potential enemy, to the extent that they feel that they may be shot and killed by anyone whom they have occasion to stop and question, to that extent they cease to be "cops on the beat." They become, instead, an armed force that may act in opposition to the very people they are sworn to protect and serve.

How long do these developments have to continue until it is no longer easy to distinguish the local police department from a military garrison that is stationed in your city? How far will we then have come from the cherished American tradition, taught to every child, that the policeman is your neighbor and your best friend?

4.   *The cost of large numbers of children and adolescents lost, especially in our inner cities.*

Many children are lost because they work in the cocaine trade. They start young, when they are nine or ten years old. They do it because there is money, big money to be made. To them, it seems like a profession. There are entry-level positions and more advanced positions. They work their way up the ladder in the same way that others do in the mainstream business world.

The difference is that the work is criminal in nature. However, if you are culturally disadvantaged, if you have two strikes against you to begin with, if you feel that you have no way to get ahead if you follow the normal, traditional routes, then the fact that your "profession" is illegal will be of little concern to you. You will tune out and be unresponsive to the extolling of traditional values by parents and teachers. The virtues of achievement via hard work and education are not likely to be as appealing as the easy money to be made on the street.

One of the costs of the unsolved cocaine problem is the tragic isolation of many inner-city young people from mainstream American values.

5. *The public health costs of increased transmission of diseases like AIDS.*

In some of our cities intravenous drug users now are the major spreaders of the HIV virus, the cause of AIDS. The spread occurs because addicts share the needles used to inject drugs. In this process diseased blood can be transferred from an infected individual to a healthy individual. In fact, there is probably no more direct way of transferring the virus than this. Illicit drug users have been sharing needles for a long time, but cocaine use has increased their number.

These not-so-willingly discussed costs are among the most important burdens the cocaine problem puts upon society. They have continued to increase in spite of the strenuous efforts we have made to curb cocaine use. The basic reason is that our thinking has been held captive by our slogans. We have been unable to stand back and look at the problem objectively and dispassionately. We have not been able to examine some basic aspects of cause and effect. It is only recently that important, distinguished voices have asked how much of these hidden costs are directly the fault of the drug and how much is due to our attempts to solve the problem. For the most part these questioning voices have been dismissed as being misguided. No matter how bad the problem becomes, no matter how many policy initiatives have failed to stem the tide of cocaine abuse, no matter how much money has been spent with little to show for it, since we are dealing with drug abuse, we are told, let's keep on doing what we've been doing until it works.

We have been reasoning exactly like this since 1914, when the Harrison Narcotic Act was passed by Congress. That act was the first serious attempt in the United States to control the use of dangerous drugs by the enactment of prohibitive legislation. It is of more than passing interest to note that cocaine, while not being a narcotic, was one of the drugs targeted by the legislation. This inaccurate classification of cocaine as a narcotic is an early example of the tendency to simplify the problem of drug abuse. The implementation of the Harrison Narcotic Act, with its emphasis on prohibition, set the pattern for all future legislative approaches to the drug-abuse problem.

These approaches have not been effective. Drug abuse is not less of a problem today than it was in 1914—not even the heroin problem, the primary target of the legislation.

As the problem worsens, and as the number of cocaine users continues to increase, the hidden costs of cocaine mount in direct proportion. These hidden costs are a direct result of having failed to solve the drug problem before it became so bad. To make matters worse, the street crime, the background violence and the disillusionment with the system are all *unnecessary* costs of cocaine use. They are unnecessary because they would not exist if the problem had been solved sooner.

Furthermore, as the hidden costs of cocaine mount, it becomes increasingly difficult for those in authority to change their thinking about them. To do so would be to inquire more critically into cause and effect. It would require examining the possibility that their programs were partially responsible for the deteriorating situation. Instead of this kind of reexamination we are assured that cocaine is a problem of drug abuse and can be dealt with like we deal with all drugs of abuse.

But cocaine, as should be evident by now, is not just another drug. Nor is any drug of the future beyond cocaine likely to be just another drug. Coping with the drug threat in a post-cocaine era will require the abandonment of the simplistic thinking that has characterized our efforts until now. If this is not done, it is extremely unlikely that future attempts to deal with the problem will be any more successful than past efforts have been.

But there is another reason why it is crucial to modify our thinking about cocaine and pleasure-producing, post-cocaine drugs. That reason has to do with the price-of-success costs that are likely to be associated with an uncritical application of "more-of-the-same" thinking. These costs are rarely brought before the American people, yet they represent the most chilling of all of the costs associated with the cocaine epidemic. They must be brought up front in any discussion of how to meet the challenge of cocaine.

How Do I Know If I Want to Buy It If You Won't Tell Me How Much It Costs?

In the case of a public health problem like AIDS, placing a price tag on efforts to solve it is relatively straightforward. The costs are found in treatment, prevention, research and education. While estimating these costs may be subject to error, no one has doubts about where the costs come from.

Cocaine, however, is an entirely different matter. Drug abuse, including the abuse of cocaine, is not really treated by our government as a public health problem. It should be, and at times you will hear people talk as if it is, but the reality is usually quite different. Drug abuse in the United States is largely considered to be a problem for the criminal justice system. Because of this, costs incurred in finding solutions to the problem are not as readily determined and not as evident to the public. This is unfortunate because looking at these price-of-success costs may lead us to question their acceptability. We may find that the costs are too high. Furthermore, we may conclude that the vast expenditures have not, and probably will not, yield the desired results.

One thing needs to be made very clear in this context. The poor return on the money invested in the "war on drugs" is not the fault of the frontline troops fighting that war. The local police, the FBI, DEA agents, county sheriffs, U.S. marshals and employees of numerous other agencies have worked heroically to reduce drug abuse. They have fought tirelessly, and many of them have died in the struggle. The problem is that these foot soldiers have been told that they are fighting a war on drugs. *In reality, they are waging war against the biological nature of man.*

In a war on drugs, the objective is to reduce both the supply of drug coming into the country and the domestic demand for it. And so the numbers pile up in headline after headline: "Six hundred pounds of cocaine seized." "Twenty members of drug ring rounded up." Numbers like these are the "body count" of the politicians and the administrators who are in the forefront of the war on drugs. And like all body counts, they can be misused. In the quest for better numbers, logistics supplants strategic thinking. A concentration on the body count tends to focus attention on isolated skirmishes, on firefights that rage at one point or another on a global battlefield. The overall picture fades away. Most important, we can lose sight of the very nature of the larger conflict in the heat of battles waged to make the numbers look better.

In reality, the frontline troops are not engaged in a simple battle to come out on the good side of the numbers game. They are engaged in a campaign to stamp out of the human species, in the space of a lifetime, what evolution has built into the species over millions of years. The pleasure produced by drugs like cocaine is sought by some people in ways that are similar to the universal search for sexual gratification. There is a lesson to be drawn from this comparison. While societies have long recognized the desirability of attempting to *regulate* sexual activity, no viable society has ever considered trying to *abolish* it. Trying to stamp out the use of chemical switches to turn on brain pleasure centers may prove to be at least as difficult as trying to get people to stop being sexual creatures.

This is not to say that drug use cannot be curtailed. It can be. The question to ask is, "What means are to be employed in achieving this result?" Our immediate concern here is to examine the costs that would be incurred by society of winning this war if we continue to employ the same means that we have always employed. Given the real nature of the war, what are we willing to spend to win it?

The fly-in-the-ointment is the notion of costs. When the topic is cocaine abuse and its eradiction by coercive means, no one has yet conveyed to the American public in a realistic way what the costs are likely to be. Granted that enormous benefits would accrue to society if cocaine use were eradicated. Unfortunately, no one has ever given the American public a clear understanding of the costs of achieving those benefits through a reliance on coercive methods. It has been, and will continue to be, a tragic mistake to embark on this kind of program without a thorough examination of these costs.

What Is the Price of Success?

The price tag of the latest phase of the War on Drugs was announced in September of 1989 to be on the order of $7.9 billion. Most of it was spent on the construction of new prisons and on an increase in law enforcement efforts to interdict supply and discourage demand. That is a lot of money. But not too much if indeed it gets the job done, and if that $7.9 million represents the actual cost of the program. To be generous, it could even be said that twice that amount would be a bargain, if there were no hidden costs. A little bit of thought, however, suggests that such dollar costs are only a weak reflection of such a program's true cost to society. The reasons can be seen by examining in more detail the two emphases of the program, supply and demand.

Most dispassionate observers of the cocaine scene would agree that the interdiction of supply is not likely to be very successful. It is extremely improbable that the amount of cocaine coming into this country can ever be reduced to a level that would make it difficult for people to find. Similar programs have been repeatedly tried in the past, most notably with marijuana and heroin, and they have failed miserably. In the early 1970s, most of the heroin coming into this country originated in Turkey. The solution was to target the opium poppy growers in that country and dry up the supply. Opium growers can be targeted in several ways. One of the more ingenious methods at the time was to pay the peasant growers (and the Turkish government) about $35 million not to grow the plants, and to help them to grow other crops. This amount of money resulted in a ban on opium growing in Turkey that lasted only about two years. Furthermore, as pressure increased in Turkey the opium business simply drifted to more hospitable shores. Mexico, for example, became a big producer. When things got too hot in Mexico, production shifted to Southeast Asia. It is still there.

(Additionally, this type of strategy does not work very well. The price of crude drugs at the source is only a very small fraction of the price of the drug on the street, about 1 percent in the case of marijuana and heroin and 4 percent in the case of cocaine. There is a lot of room to maneuver in making a profit in illegal drugs.)

There is a lesson here, of course. Poor people will raise cash crops as long as someone will pay them for their efforts. Put yourself in their shoes. You are eking out a marginal existence in a third-world country, barely able to make ends meet and feed your family. Someone comes along and offers to pay you well to grow opium plants or marijuana plants or cocaine plants. You are probably not going to lose much sleep over the fact that the fruit of your labors causes difficulty to some rich American thousands of miles away from you.

(Incidentally, one of the unintended results of a similar campaign to discourage foreign growth of marijuana—that is to reduce supply—was to increase production of the plant in the United States. The home-grown variety, incidentally, is much more potent than the foreign-grown ever was. Americans now grow some of the best marijuana in the world. Another "benefit" of this approach was to make our National Forests a little more dangerous for hikers and nature lovers. Several of these innocent people have been shot or booby-trapped by marijuana growers bent on protecting their little patch in the free enterprise system.)

The focus in 1991 on the coca growers in Colombia can be expected to yield similar results. Coca can be, will be and is being grown in other locations. In South America alone, there are about 2,500,000 square miles of territory where the coca plant will grow well. About 700 square miles are currently used to grow the plant. Take whatever portion of the $7.9 billion that is dedicated to local interdiction and multiply it by about 3,600. That's a beginning estimate of how much it would cost even to *start* interdiction efforts in that continent alone.

Furthermore, the flow of cocaine into this country is unlikely to change much as a result of this type of interdiction effort. These tactics are not even likely to cause a long-term increase in the street price of the drug. During the past decade, for example, as interdiction efforts have grown, the wholesale price of a kilogram of cocaine has dropped some 80 percent. At the same time, the purity of cocaine sold on the streets of our cities has increased to around 60 percent.

But multiplying the apparent cost of this type of program by three or four thousand does not reveal the most important hidden cost of this approach. More important long range costs stem from effects of the program that are studiously ignored by policy makers, effects that include:

- Depriving local peasants of their main source of income, in many cases making the difference between an adequate and an impoverished standard of living.
- Stimulating, as a result, a hatred of Yankee imperialism that can drive these same peasants into the arms of revolutionary political parties. Some observers see evidence of this process already benefiting parties like the Shining Path in Peru.
- Increased involvement of American military forces on the ground as drug-revolutionary armies become more difficult for the local government to control.

- The possible emergence of retaliatory terrorist attacks by these same groups on Americans at home and everywhere in the world.

The costs of success of a foreign policy increasingly driven by a poorly conceived war on drugs are never pointed out to the American people. These costs represent a potential political disaster for the United States.

What about the other side of the ledger? Maybe the outlook is better for controlling domestic demand. The obvious way to do this is to police the situation more vigorously and to arrest more people. But what is an increase in policing to be compared with? What does it cost to do the policing at the current level? Most important, since resources are limited, what are the implications of this increased focus on drug consumers for policing other crimes? Here are some current costs that are not usually revealed when the citizen is asked to pay more for a beefed-up war on drugs:

- In 1989 the Federal Government spent about $4 *billion* enforcing drug laws. The 1990 figure was on the order of $5.8 billion. These figures do not include costs at the state and local levels.
- At the state and local level, about one-fifth of the investigative budget of law enforcement agencies is earmarked for drug enforcement.
- Federal government money spent on drug enforcement between 1981 and 1987 increased more than three times. The amount requested for 1991 is an increase to $6.3 billion from the $4 billion spent in 1989.

As more and more law enforcement resources are devoted to the drug problem, less and less attention is directed to other crimes. The cost of success is that local police have less and less time to investigate, solve and punish rapists, armed robbers, kidnappers, hold-up artists, perpetrators of assault and battery, muggers, extortionists and other criminals. As the emphasis on drug offenses increases, you can expect the police will more often be unable to respond to your call for help in timely fashion. If a larger proportion of resources and personnel is dedicated to tracking drug users, fewer officers will be available to respond to your report of a crime in progress in your neighborhood.

Here are some additional figures that are not widely understood:

- The proportion of prison inmates jailed for drug offenses rises yearly. In federal prisons they will amount to about 50 percent of all prisoners in ten to fifteen years.
- In 1988, state and local governments spent at least $2 *billion* to imprison drug offenders.
- Given the size of these numbers, it is important to realize that the number of people arrested represents only about 2 percent of 40,000,000 Americans estimated to have used drugs illegally last year.

Imprisoning people who use drugs will certainly remove some drug users from the streets. The cost of doing so, however, would bankrupt the country. Besides, what kind of a country is it that would put forty million of its citizens in jail? What is the cost of success of a war that incarcerates one-fifth of its population?

There are additional costs of success that are even more disturbing. If domestic demand is to be reduced by incarcerating drug users, there must be some way to catch them. One of the ways that has been suggested is mandatory drug testing for everyone. Consider some of the logistical questions involved. When should such testing begin, that is to say, at what age? If we are to use testing as a deterrent, perhaps logic demands that the process begin early in life, so that the deterrent effect is felt even before the individual has had much occasion to come into contact with drugs. So one possibility is to begin testing when children are five or six years old. This is not fanciful. Drug use is increasingly common among school-age children. They are routinely exposed to it as early as junior high school, and in some cases even earlier.

Since one test is certainly not sufficient, we must determine how often we should test if we are to have any assurance that the citizenry is free of drugs. If we begin at an early age, tests could be conducted at the beginning of each school year, or perhaps each semester. The process could be continued through the college years and on into the workplace. Perhaps a clean bill of health on a drug screen could be required for admission to an institution of higher learning or as part of a job application.

Finally, we will have to decide where such testing is to be done. Consider the question of taking urine specimens for analysis. Perhaps we can arrange for it to be done in the privacy of your home. If not, surely it can be carried out in the workplace, with proper safeguards (urine monitors?) to insure that people do not cheat in donating their urine. Or maybe the urine samples can be taken at the police station, even perhaps at three o'clock in the morning, following an unanticipated knock at your door.

If you say that it can't happen here, you're wrong. Serious voices have already been raised suggesting that, *when it's a question of drug abuse,* it might be acceptable to forego some of the liberties guaranteed you under the Bill Of Rights.

There is another way that drug users can be apprehended. It's called *informing.* That means turning in your friends, your neighbors, your children or your parents. It means turning in your business associates or (a more interesting possibility) your competitors. We can become a nation of eavesdroppers, spies, and stool-pigeons, all with the encouragement of the government, and all in the name of a drug-free society.

Simply put, to remove drug users from the scene, to remove the demand factor, would require turning the country into a police state in which individual liberty would disappear.

How to Lose Both the Battle and the War

So how bad is it? What is the scope of the cocaine problem?

The scope is defined by the war that is waged. In the War on Drugs, in a world of cocaine and the future beyond cocaine, it is not the stated costs that matter. Not in the long run. The costs that matter in the long run are the hidden costs and the costs of success. It is the very nature of these costs to remain hidden until it is too late. Too late, that is, because the bill will have come due. The tab will have been paid. There will be no way to go back and ask for a reaccounting. There will be no way to have the bill reexamined to see if it should have been paid.

On the other hand, we can bring these costs into the open and face them squarely. We may conclude, in fact, that *some* drug testing is necessary. In these cases we should not embark upon such programs lightly. Rather, we should demand rigorous demonstrations that any proposed testing is crucial to the well-being of the community and nation. We should resist the imposition of testing programs that are only the whims of people in positions of power. In similar fashion, all of us should be willing to report a crime when we see it. The trick is to avoid defining crime in such a way that we are pushed ever farther into monitoring the private lives of our friends and neighbors.

If we are not very careful, we put ourselves at great risk. The ultimate cost of the war on cocaine is likely to be a fundamental change in the American understanding of democracy. The ultimate cost of the war will be an erosion of individual liberty. The waging of the war will mark the beginning of an intrusion of government into the private lives of individuals that will make a mockery of constitutional guarantees of freedom from self-incrimination and protection from unreasonable search and seizure. The war on cocaine will condemn our children to a world that our fathers would not recognize, a world in which their every move, their every transaction, is compiled and monitored by government computers. If we are not careful, the war on cocaine will begin the process whereby the government comes to be the master of the common man rather than his servant.

Chapter 8

How Bad Can It Get?
What Lies Beyond Cocaine?

Imagine a future like the following:

Neuroscientists have made enormous strides in understanding the details of how drugs work on individual nerve cells. They know which cells are the natural target of a given drug, and they know the particular part of the cell that is affected by the drug. That is, they know the site and mechanism of action of the drug.

Simple chemicals are available that can be used in the manufacture of a large variety of drugs. These chemicals are abundant and cheap. They can be used to make large quantities of drugs, from scratch, with no dependence on plant sources like coca, marijuana or opium poppy.

These chemicals are so common that they are in everyday use in thousands of manufacturing processes around the world. They are chemicals that are basic to the manufacture of countless common goods and products that are indispensable to everyday life.

The process of making drugs from these chemicals is incredibly simple. Easy-to-follow recipes are widely circulated showing how to use these chemicals to make potent mind-altering drugs.

It is not an easy matter to pass laws outlawing these drugs

because too much is known about the relationship between the structure of the drug and its mechanism of action in the brain. Whenever a specific drug is outlawed, the illicit drug maker can make a new drug by modifying a portion of the outlawed drug. He modifies, however, only those portions of the drug that are not crucial to the effect that the drug produces. He leaves the important part of the molecule unchanged. If this new drug is outlawed, he simply repeats the process and makes another new drug. This process can be repeated almost indefinitely.

The drug maker's activity cannot be easily controlled by restricting the availability of the basic chemicals. This would lead to unacceptable increases in their cost and in the cost of the legitimate products that are made from them. These products are in such widespread use that to do without them, or to artificially inflate their price, would produce an unacceptable decline in the standard of living of the entire population.

Because of the level of scientific knowledge, it is increasingly likely that some, perhaps many, of the drugs produced will be much more addicting than cocaine.

Welcome to the future. It is now.

America's Greatest Cottage Industry

Making drugs is easy. By 1970, in fact, home recipes for making a number of common drugs were readily available on the street. This do-it-yourself approach to drug manufacture blossomed in the mid-1970s as an unintended by-product of the attempt by law enforcement agencies to stem an amphetamine epidemic.

Amphetamines had worked their way into a drug culture that, at the outset, centered on marijuana and LSD. The original participants in this drug culture, the hippies and flower children of the 1960s, did not welcome this new drug. Nor did they particularly care for the type of person who was associated with this drug. The slogan "SPEED KILLS" was coined by the flower children to indicate that amphetamine was a very dangerous drug. But of perhaps greater significance to the earlier members of the "Turn on, tune in, and drop out" generation, it could be destructive to their community. With its tendency to produce paranoia and violence, amphetamine was seen to be hostile to group harmony and well-being.

As the 1970s wore on, amphetamine became the number one drug problem in California. The dimensions of the problem were appalling. So, too, were some of the social aspects of the increased street popularity of the drug. Unscrupulous physicians, called "script writers," could be found who would write prescriptions for amphetamines on the slimmest of pretexts. Compliasant pharmacists could always be found to fill them. Finally, a public outcry demanded that something be done about it. Law enforcement priorities were accordingly shifted to focus on this latest aspect of the drug scourge.

As part of the effort to stem the tide, attention was directed toward putting an end to the diversion of legal amphetamines to illicit street use. The idea was to make it more difficult to obtain amphetamine by constricting the source of supply. This law enforcement effort had three major effects: legally manufactured amphetamines did, in fact, show up in much smaller quantities for street use; hard-up, hard-core amphetamine users discovered cocaine, initiating the whirlwind cocaine problem, which has not yet abated; and enterprising drug merchants discovered that they could easily make their own amphetamines to cover the shortfall in legally manufactured drugs. This third effect is the one of interest here.

Do It Yourself: A Venerable American Tradition

Speed Labs. The phrase is now a part of the modern American vocabulary. It refers to the illicit manufacture of amphetamine that will be sold illegally on the street. Speed labs are a ubiquitous part of the American scene. They proliferated as a direct result of stepped-up law enforcement efforts directed toward reducing the illegal use of legally manufactured amphetamines. The harder it became to get legally manufactured amphetamines, the greater was the incentive to produce them illegally. American enterpreneurship, sensing profits to be made, rose to this challenge of diminished supply.

Speed Labs. They have become even more common of late. They satisfy a market that feels under some pressure as a result of law enforcement concentration on cocaine. There is a kind of buckets-in-the-well relationship between these two drugs. As law enforcement priorities shift and concentrate on eliminating one of them, users tend to increase their use of the other. They are both central-nervous-system stimulants. Their subjective effects are similar enough that the devoted user of one has no difficulty using the other when his preferred drug is hard to get.

Speed labs and the illicit manufacture of drugs provide the first insight into the world of the future, when drugs even more destructive than cocaine may be a part of life in the United States.

When Is a Rose Not a Rose?

There are many words in use on the street to describe amphetamine and related drugs: speed, crank, crystal, crystal-meth. The two major drugs referred to by all of these names are amphetamine and methamphetamine. Methamphetamine is virtually identical to amphetamine from a chemical standpoint, having a methyl group substituted for one of the hydrogen atoms of the amphetamine molecule. And both of these compounds are strikingly similar to dopamine (DA) and to a related neurotransmitter, norepinephrine (NE). The chemical formulas of these compounds are shown in Figure 8.1.

Drugs that are closely related in their chemical architecture tend to produce similar effects in the body. This similarity is useful to the

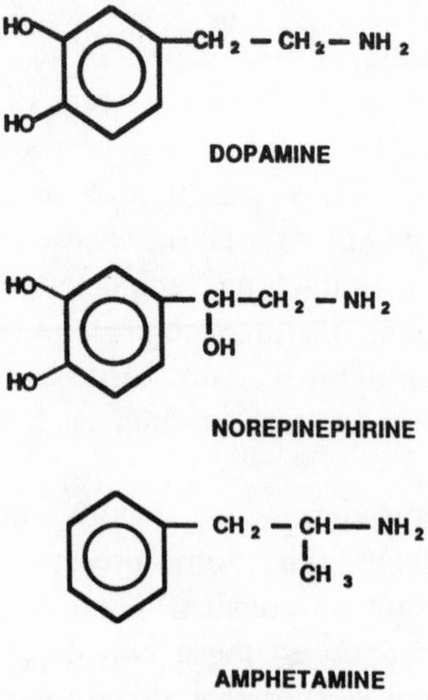

Fig. 8.1 Chemical formulas showing similarity in structure of dopamine, norepinephrine and amphetamine

designer of drugs. If he wants to make a drug that produces a given effect, he does not have to start from scratch. In many cases, he can look to existing drugs that produce the same or similar effects and start from there.

The drugs, although similar, are, in fact, different drugs. Two drugs are not the same drug unless they are identical in the placement of all of their constituent atoms. The substitution of $-CH_3$ for $-H$ makes methamphetamine a different drug than amphetamine.

But, you say, "Well, they may be different drugs if you want to split hairs. But their effects are so similar that they might as well be called the same drug." And there you have put your finger on one very large problem for a society contemplating drug abuse problems in the future, that future beyond cocaine.

Because they are, in fact, different drugs, legal statements applied to one do not automatically apply to the other, even though everyone might be willing to concede that their effects are similar. In order to classify a drug for legal purposes, it is necessary to know what drug you are talking about. The only way to do that is to specify its structure, that is, the arrangements of its constituent atoms in three-dimensional space. By definition, then, drugs of dissimilar atomic architecture are different drugs.

If you were in the business of making illegal drugs, this distinction would not be lost on you. You would probably say to yourself something like the following:

"Let's see now. There are many, many modifications that I can make to the amphetamine molecule, any one of which produces a new drug which is technically not amphetamine. Hence, it is in principle not an illegal substance. It should be possible, too, that some of those potential modifications will produce a drug which is legally not an amphetamine yet which has the same or similar effects. Such a drug, until it comes within the purview of the law, can be sold legally to all of those people out there who are into amphetamine. That is a large market. Let me, therefore, go about my creative endeavors."

If you have reasoned like this, you have just invented *designer drugs*.

Because the makers of designer drugs or, more technically, analog drugs have reasoned like this, the federal government recently passed legislation in an attempt to deal with the problem. In 1985, emergency provisions of the law were invoked to place some opiate analogs under federal control. Since 1986, the controlled substance label can be applied to all analogs of drugs which are classified as controlled substances.

Nevertheless, designer drugs merit serious consideration. They are a relatively new phenomenon, having made their first appearance a few years ago with the drug "Ecstasy." Other drugs like "Eve" soon followed. The problems that such drugs pose for society are enormous. In the future beyond cocaine these problems may become insurmountable. The reasons for this possibility will be easier to see if designer drugs are viewed against the backdrop of legitimate drug manufacture. The legal production of drugs will, in the future, guarantee that the makers of designer drugs will be able to turn out substances that are even more addicting than those available today.

Mainstream Drug Manufacture: All of the Elves Are Busy

So the focus shifts, for the moment, from the makers of illicit drugs to the activities of another group of drug designers. These are people who are equally interested in the possibilities of modifying known drug structures, or of inventing new drug structures, in order to accomplish well-formulated objectives. It is their lifework. They get paid for it. These designers are, of course, the pharmacologists, the scientists who design virtually all of the drugs in use today. A look at this industry will shed considerable light on some of the problems that our society will confront in the years ahead.

Pharmaceutical firms, drug companies, are profitable only when they have a product that the public is anxious to buy. For this reason they spend enormous sums of money on the development of new and innovative drugs, drugs, in other words, that will give them a greater market share, a greater piece of the pie, a leg up on the competition.

This process of research and development produces an enormous number of new drugs. Most of them never reach the marketplace simply because they offer no competitive advantage in the quest for the consumer's dollar. Either they represent no therapeutic advance or other products are already available that will do the job at less cost. Nevertheless, vast amounts are spent each year in the quest for new drugs, because the financial stakes are so high.

There is nothing wrong here. Society can benefit from such

scientific pursuits. New and improved medicines hold the promise of treating and perhaps even curing many of the diseases that today are untreatable. New drugs have the potential for turning tragedy into triumph, despair into hope.

A society that is concerned with the future, and what it holds with respect to drug abuse, can learn a lot by examining the process by which these discoveries are made and the scientific procedures that govern the quest.

Some major discoveries have been made, of course, by accident. Librium is a case in point. It nearly missed seeing the light of day because it was almost thrown away. And without Librium there would have been no Valium. And Valium is perhaps the single most prescribed medication in the United States.

The story goes like this. A chemist named L. H. Sternbach was working at the University of Cracow in Poland in the years just before World War II. He was engaged in the synthesis of cyclic or ring compounds for reasons that had nothing to do with drugs. Forced to leave Poland because of the Nazi threat, he found himself after the war working as a research director for Roche Labs in Western Europe.

Sternbach had taken some of his earlier-synthesized compounds with him to the West. Since he was now in the employ of a drug firm, he did the normal thing. He tested his compounds to see if any of them had any interesting biological activity. There were a number of the compounds to be examined, and the testing was done methodically, one by one. All but one of the compounds had been tested without discovering anything of any biological interest when the process had to be abandoned because other laboratory work commanded a higher priority. The remaining original compound sat on the shelf until a few years later. It was rediscovered while the lab was undergoing a kind of housecleaning, and for the sake of completeness it was tested for biological activity.

The rest, as they say, is history. The compound is now called Librium, and it proved to be a gold mine for Roche. The company is sometimes referred to among drug researchers as "The House That Librium Built."

Numerous other examples of this kind of serendipity can be cited in the history of drug development and research.

- The psychedelic properties of lysergic acid diethylamide (LSD) were stumbled upon accidentally by Albert Hofmann in Switzerland, in 1943, when he inadvertently ingested some of the compound while working at the lab bench. He wasn't deliberately trying to find psychedelic drugs. He had been working for several years with ergot, a fungus that grows on grain, synthesizing compounds that were similar to known stimulants.
- The phenothiazine drugs that are used to treat schizophrenia first came to attention as biological agents in the mid-1950s when they were used to potentiate surgical anesthesia. They had originally been synthesized in the German dye industry in the late nineteenth century.
- Meprobamate, or Equanil, one of the first tranquilizers, was the result of a search for an antibiotic that would be useful in treating penicillin-resistant bacterial diseases. The search began with the modification of insecticides.

The stories make good telling. Perhaps they are even a source of comfort to those of us whose fortunes have not been as bountiful as we might have hoped. Good luck, after all, may be just around the corner. In the present context, however, the histories are useful because, by standing in stark contrast to the more routine, day-to-day work of science, they help to illustrate the systematic and methodical way in which drug research is currently carried out.

Times have changed since the days of Niemann and Freud. Chemistry has changed, especially biochemistry, the chemistry of living organisms. Neuroanatomy and neurophysiology have changed. Genetics today would be unrecognizable to the geneticists of a century ago. These and other fields of study like psychology, pharmacology and physics have fused today into a scientific discipline that did not even exist when Niemann isolated cocaine from the coca plant.

The field is neuroscience. Its practitioners come from many scientific disciplines. They are bound together, and their work takes on a unity, because of a shared interest in arriving at the fullest possible understanding of the workings of the nervous system, especially the workings of the human brain. In pursuit of this end, they have at their disposal an armamentarium of skills and techniques that allow penetration deep into the secrets of the brain and mind of man. Their work has yielded exciting insights into several of the more perplexing mental disorders of humankind. It holds the promise of further discoveries that may eliminate pathological conditions that have bedeviled our species for centuries.

All of these skills are brought into play in the search for drugs that have the human brain as their site of action. The neuropharmacologist, a scientist who studies drugs that work on the nervous system, has been trained in the most modern methods of neuroscience research. He has a detailed knowledge of the structure and function of the brain. He is a pioneer in the development of new knowledge about the way in which brain cells process information. The neuropharmacologist develops and uses drugs as chemical probes.

How does he go about his business? In what particulars is his work with drugs different from the work performed by his intellectual predecessors of a few years ago? And how does this change in approach relate to drug addiction, designer drugs and the world of the future?

Start With a Good Plan and Pay Attention to the Details

Perhaps of greatest importance is the modern scientist's recognition that there is a definite relationship between the structure of a drug and the actions that it can produce in the brain. Drugs like cocaine, amphetamine, opiates and tranquilizers produce their characteristic effects because of this structure-activity relationship. That is, the activity of a drug in the brain (and the effects it produces) depends on its structure (its chemical architecture). Because the scientist has greater knowledge of the fine-grain details of this relationship, drug development is no longer a haphazard or random affair. It is a deliberate search in which selected aspects of drug structure can be systematically modified and varied in an effort to find new drugs that produce desired effects with greater degrees of precision.

An analogy may be useful here. A chemist builds molecules much as a carpenter builds a house. He starts with an overall plan, as the carpenter does with a blueprint, which tells him, in effect, where he wants to end up. His overall plan, in other words, tells him what the molecule will look like. Then, just as the builder puts the house together a piece at a time, working first on the foundation and then on the walls, the scientist constructs his molecule one portion at a time. He will first link atoms together to make the basic "backbone" (the foundation) of the molecule. He will then add components as he works toward the final product he has envisioned.

The analogy can be pushed still further. Some elements of a house are essential if the structure is to be recognized as a house. There must be walls, a roof, doors and a few other basic features. Other elements, however, are not essential to the definition of a house. There may be a conservatory or a garage, and still the structure qualifies as a house. Furthermore, an almost limitless amount of variation is possible in the constructional details of the building's components. One bath or two? Atrium or foyer? One-car garage or two? These components can be varied almost endlessly without changing the basic character of the structure.

The same is true of chemical molecules, including drugs. All of the various drugs that exist can be thought of as falling into different categories based on their architecture. (There are numerous other ways of classifying drugs. Some are important organizational schemes, like the one which is examined in the next chapter.) Figuratively speaking, some drugs are town houses, and others are ranch houses. Some are Georgian and others are French provincial. Within each of these categories of architecture, however, there are many possible ways of varying the structure without destroying the basic plan.

Consider an example directly related to the topic of this book. Cocaine can be classified as a local anesthetic. It is no longer used for this purpose to the extent that it once was because other, less troublesome local anesthetics have been developed. They have familiar names like Novocaine and Lidocaine. The interesting thing is that most of these other local anesthetics have chemical structures that are *very* similar to the structure of cocaine.

The central fact is that their structural similarity to cocaine makes these drugs effective local anesthetics. A certain basic molecular structure, call it French provincial, guarantees that the drug serves as a local anesthetic. A Georgian edifice would not do the job.

But why are drugs like Novocaine and Lidocaine more widely

used than cocaine? Why, with few exceptions, have they replaced cocaine in clinical medicine? Simply because they do not stimulate the CNS and produce euphoria in the same way that cocaine does. Consequently they are less likely to be abused. And why do they not stimulate the CNS as much? Because, while similar, they are not identical in structure to cocaine. By retaining the parts of the molecule that serve to define it as being, say, of the French provincial type, the drug designer has preserved the local anesthetic character of the molecule. That is, local anesthetic action depends on this basic part of the molecule. The parts of the molecule that have been modified are those that have, so to speak, changed the appearance of some of the rooms of the house without modifying its basic French provincial character.

By the same token, the modifications in structure seem to have made the molecule a "better" local anesthetic. But, some caution is necessary in making this appraisal. The noncocaine anesthetics are not as potent as cocaine in relieving pain. Milligram for milligram, cocaine is a better pain reliever. Drugs like Novocaine are "better" local anesthetics than cocaine only in that they do not produce the undesirable effects of CNS stimulation and euphoria. And that, after all, is why they are important.

If, by manipulating chemical structure, it is possible to make cocainelike drugs that do not produce the euphoria that cocaine does, should it not be possible to make other alterations that produce even more euphoria than is found with cocaine? Never mind the problem of local anesthesia. Concentrate on the CNS effects themselves. Concentrate on the very effects of cocaine that make it undesirable in medical use. Then create a new drug in which these effects are even more prominent.

But wait a minute. Why would anyone want to do this? Don't drugs cause enough trouble already? Why look for drugs that outperform cocaine in their ability to produce pleasurable brain stimulation? Several motivations come to mind. The most obvious are those influencing the maker of designer drugs. If he can produce a new drug that is, at least in the short run, not an illicit substance, he has a product that poses fewer risks for him. If, in addition, he stumbles upon a drug that produces a better high, then his market and his profits are likely to increase. One motivation, in other words, is greed.

More important, however, are the motives of the scientists. Drugs for these people are tools. They are *chemical probes* of the brain. The motive here is perhaps the strongest of all, curiosity. With curiosity goes the thrill of discovery. If that discovery happens to be important and the scientist makes it before anyone else does, well, then, throw in the desire for fame as another motive. These powerful motives drive legions of researchers.

What is the likely outcome of all this activity? We will see an increasing number of new and better drugs. Among these will almost certainly be drugs that provide improved keys to unlock the pleasure centers of the brain. These drugs will produce greater euphoria than does crack, and they will be even more addicting.

Once again, welcome to the future. Welcome to the future. . . .

Beyond Cocaine

The vision can be a bit frightening. There are thousands of bright, creative scientists toiling away in hundreds of pharmaceutical laboratories around the world, all engaged in the search for better and better drugs. "Better" here means more specific, more selective drugs that do exactly what the drug manufacturer wants them to do, with a minimum of unwanted side effects. As I've indicated, the motivation to produce these drugs is strong, and the payoff for finding a successful product is great. The quest is not likely to end soon.

Factor in, furthermore, the thousands of basic research scientists at work in universities around the globe. Ninety-nine percent of all of the scientists who have ever lived are alive today. Each and every one of them is engaged in an unrelenting push to expand the frontiers of scientific knowledge. Among these frontiers is one of the most challenging and exciting of all, the human brain.

Nothing like today's knowledge explosion has been seen before in the entire history of the human race. Increasingly fine-grain detail about the workings of the brain is being reported on a daily basis. The brain is a chemical machine surrendering its secrets at an accelerating rate: new information about the information-processing capabilities of neurons, fresh discoveries of the subtle means by which one neuron passes information to another, clearer insight into the workings of these cells in health and disease.

Among the secrets yielded up by the brain will undoubtedly be found those leading to an increasingly sophisticated understanding of the mechanisms of pleasure. A lot of people are interested in these mechanisms. And why not? After all, information about the way in which the brain is able to construct the experience of pleasure out of the activity of its neurons bears directly on the most fundamental questions that can be asked about how the brain controls behavior. Among the information about pleasure that is waiting to be discovered is knowledge of how to control it better by chemical means.

A Closer Look at Pleasure

While it may at first seem paradoxical, the high degree of complexity in the brain's reward circuitry increases the likelihood that drugs can be designed to activate it with a greater degree of selectivity than cocaine does today. It goes without saying that such new drugs would have greater potential to wreak havoc in our society than do the currently available drugs of abuse. A more complete look at the brain's pleasure circuitry, as it is known today, can provide a useful springboard for an intriguing, if somewhat anxiety-provoking, look into the future.

The concept of pleasure centers in the brain has developed in recent years into the idea of pleasure *circuits*. This latter way of speaking is much more consistent with current scientific understanding of the mechanisms of pleasure. The experience of pleasure does not seem to depend as much on a particular, circumscribed small area of the brain as it does on increased activity in certain circuits. Granted, the aggregate of these circuits, insofar as they connect specific brain regions that lie in proximity to one another, could be referred to as a pleasure center. Keeping the multicomponent aspect in mind, however, will highlight the cellular complexity that underlies the experience of pleasure. This complexity, in turn, suggests the possibility of fine-tuned intervention in the brain's interpretation of pleasurable events.

Figure 8.2 illustrates a currently popular conception of what may be involved in the pleasure circuitry of the brain. As it illustrates, feelings of intense pleasure and the experience of reward are thought

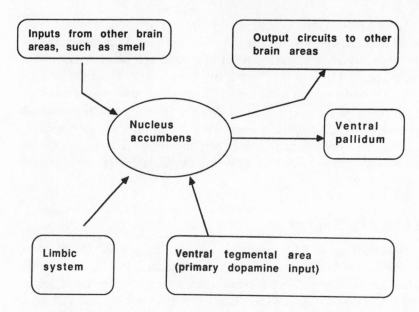

Fig. 8.2   Some major aspects of the brain's pleasure centers

to involve neural pathways that converge on the *nucleus accumbens*. Most scientists believe that increased activity in the nucleus accumbens is essential to the experience of pleasure or reward. Eating, drinking, sex and other activities are thought to be pleasurable because they produce this type of increased brain activity. They do it, of course, with varying degrees of direct connection. Electrical stimulation of some of the classical reward areas of the brain, such as those discovered by Olds, causes increases in nucleus accumbens activity by a somewhat indirect route. Cocaine, in contrast, produces such increased activity by the most direct route yet known.

The nucleus accumbens is an important component of the brain's limbic system. It is the limbic system of the brain that is critically involved in the experience and expression of emotion. Anger, love, hate, joy, ecstasy—the entire range of emotions—are all products of limbic system activity. Of course, this limbic driving of emotional states is heavily influenced by activity in other brain areas. If it were not, emotional expression would know no bounds. In humans, for example, cortical regulation of limbic arousal is crucial to that tempering of emotional expression that makes socialized group living possible.

Figure 8.2 also shows that pleasure is best thought of in terms of brain circuitry. The nucleus accumbens receives information from numerous other brain areas and sends messages to a variety of other regions of the central nervous system. The circuitry is complicated, however, and it is only beginning to be understood. It is not yet clear, for example, which of these many connections of the nucleus accumbens are of primary, and which are of secondary, importance for the experience of pleasure. Given this complexity of organization, our current understanding of the mechanisms of pleasure may be oversimplified.

For example, consider the experience of pleasure from a temporal standpoint. Pleasure is a time-bound phenomenon. It has a beginning and an end. It also has a period of time between these two points that could be called its maintenance period. Beyond the simple prolongation of neurotransmitter action discussed previously, no one has any idea at present of what the neural events are that underlie this temporal dimension of the pleasure experience. No one, that is, has yet pinpointed exactly the cellular events that mark the onset of pleasure or the events that signal its termination. And with the exception of the increased activity in the nucleus accumbens that has been discussed, scientists remain in the dark in their attempts to specify the cellular changes that are characteristic of the maintenance period of pleasure.

These questions are of more than academic interest. The temporal aspects of pleasure raise some fascinating questions about the role of drugs in producing such intense feelings. For example, drugs like cocaine obviously do a good job of initiating pleasure. Are there other drugs to be discovered that do an equally good job of maintaining pleasure once it has been initiated? Are there still other drugs that would counteract brain mechanisms that might be involved in the termination of pleasure? Is it possible that combinations of such drugs could produce and maintain high degrees of pleasure extending over prolonged periods? Questions like these suggest that in cocaine we may be looking only at the beginnings of our ability to manipulate chemically some of the most basic aspects of addictive brain mechanisms.

While the mechanisms of pleasure are complex, the importance of the nucleus accumbens seems well established. Research with animals indicates that this brain area is necessary for the animal to respond to various pleasure-inducing drugs. If the nucleus accumbens is eliminated, surgically, for example, then drugs like cocaine lose their rewarding character. Cocaine loses much of its addictive property if an individual has no nucleus accumbens.

In all of this, the neurotransmitter dopamine plays a key role. Neurons that use dopamine as a neurotransmitter make up one of the major sources of input to the nucleus accumbens. That is, the cells in the nucleus accumbens are directly stimulated by dopamine that is released onto them by presynaptic neurons. These presynaptic neurons, in turn, originate in the ventral tegmental area (VTA) of the brain. When neurons in the VTA become active they increase their release of dopamine onto the neurons in the nucleus accumbens. This event seems to be a critical first step in the initiation of the pleasurable response to stimulant drugs like cocaine.

Moreover, the rewarding effects of electrical stimulation of the classical reward sites in the brain (the sites that Olds discovered) is now thought to depend on dopamine. One of these sites is located where a group of fibers called the medial forebrain bundle runs through the lateral portion of the hypothalamus. Stimulation of this site is highly rewarding. The reason is that such stimulation causes messages to be passed to the neurons in the VTA. These messages increase the activity of the VTA neurons and cause them to increase their release of dopamine onto neurons in the nucleus accumbens.

The critical role of dopamine in mediating the effects of cocaine and of brain stimulation can easily be demonstrated. Thus, drugs are known that block the effectiveness of dopamine as a chemical messenger. Administration of these drugs disrupts the rewarding, and presumably pleasurable, effects of cocaine and of electrical stimulation of the lateral hypothalamus.

More specifically, dopamine, cocaine and the nucleus accumbens are linked in the following way. Cocaine blocks the ability of VTA neurons to reuptake the dopamine that they secrete as a neurotransmitter. The transmitter from these neurons normally activates cells in the nucleus accumbens. The increased stimulation of this nucleus that results when the chemical messenger is not taken back by the presynaptic neuron is the critical initial event in the intense pleasure that is produced by cocaine. Dopamine and the addicting power of cocaine are linked because of the action of the drug in opening this gate to the limbic system.

Receptors Revisited: How Much Pleasure Is Possible?

Small wonder, then, that one of the major thrusts of current pharmacological research is concerned with drug and neurotransmitter receptors. We have already observed that there are several different kinds of dopamine receptor. It was also pointed out that more than one kind of cocaine receptor is likely to be found in the human CNS. Indeed, scientists are not yet sure that any cocaine receptor has been unequivocally identified.

Receptor complexity and the exploitation of the brain's pleasure circuitry are related phenomena. Complex processes are subject to perturbation in complex ways. If there are several types of receptor for a given transmitter or for a given drug, it is very likely that the different sites of action mediate different neuronal responses. Or, it might be that different sites of action (i.e., different receptors) are linked to different components of the drug's effects. This implies, in turn, that drug intervention in synaptic transmission may be "fine-tuned" by designing drugs that "target" one receptor type more than another. It was this kind of design strategy that was envisioned in an earlier discussion of the development of an opiate narcotic that would relieve pain without producing addiction. The notion is that the opiate receptors which, when activated, lead to pain relief are not the same receptors whose activation produces the experience of pleasure that is presumed to underlie narcotic abuse.

In anticipating what may lie in the future of addicting drugs, the receptor question is of primary importance. The reason for this focus is apparent enough if the basic sequence of events is recalled: cocaine occupies its receptor; the reuptake of dopamine is blocked; excess stimulation of the dopamine receptor is the result. Beyond this basic sequence, however, the details become quite murky. How many dopamine receptors are there? Are they all stimulated by the excess transmitter? Do they all lead to the same response? Are all dopamine receptors equally involved in pleasure and reward? Perhaps most troubling of all is the degree of uncertainty that exists concerning the cocaine receptor itself.

Scientists are not in agreement on the number of different types of dopamine receptors. While there is disagreement on the details, most researchers would agree that dopamine receptors come in two major varieties. They are called D-1 receptors and D-2 receptors.

They represent, if you will, two different biological "locks" into which the transmitter "key" fits. The differences between these two types involve biochemical complexities which do not need to be detailed here. It is possible, nonetheless, to point out a number of their characteristics that offer thought-provoking glimpses into the future. The general idea to keep in mind is that the existence of multiple receptors for a given transmitter suggests strongly that numerous mechanisms exist for the regulation of synaptic transmission. It is exactly through the disruption of this regulation that cocaine exerts its profound effects.

Perhaps the first puzzling aspect of all of this is the idea of having two locks which are opened by the same key. Two locks, that is, that differ in truly important ways. You have to be careful in looking for a good analogy for this in the everyday world. You have certainly encountered situations where you found it useful to have several keys for the same lock. The keys are copies of one another and you regard them as being equivalent. If, conversely, you encounter a situation where two locks are opened by the same key, you regard the locks as copies of one another and interchangeable.

Multiple receptors do not exhibit quite the same interchangeability. They are more like a set of related locks, all of which are opened by a master key, but each one of which can be opened by a specific key that opens its particular lock and no other. In the receptor's case the keys are chemicals. The neurotransmitter is the master key. It opens all of the biological locks. There are other chemicals, like drugs, that can open some of these biological locks but not others. In other words, a drug may open one but not another of a set of locks, all of which are dopamine locks. The important corollary is this: the effect of a given drug depends upon which of the locks it happens to fit.

If all of this seems rather unlikely, rest assured that it is not. As a matter of fact, the separation of receptors into different types is done by the scientist in just this way. When all of the biochemical complexities are swept away, receptors are classified on the basis of which chemical keys they accept and which they reject. Dopamine receptors are all grouped together because the master key, dopamine, activates all of them. They are further classified into subtypes because some chemicals activate one subtype but have little or no effect on another subtype.

In addition to the number of receptor subtypes, major interest in this area centers on two additional topics.

1. Where are the various subtypes of receptor located?

2. What are the changes over time that receptors undergo when they are subjected to prolonged chemical stimulation by drugs?

Receptors for the neurotransmitter are found not only on the postsynaptic neuron but on the presynaptic neuron as well. That is, receptors for the neurotransmitter exist on the same neuron that releases it. Such presynaptic receptors exist on both the cell body and on the presynaptic nerve terminals themselves. When neurotransmitter is released, in other words, it stimulates not only the presynaptic neuron but also the very neuron that released it.

One of the functions of the presynaptic receptor is a kind of self-monitoring called autoregulation. For this reason, the receptors themselves are called *autoreceptors*. They influence the amount of transmitter released by monitoring the amount of neurochemical released into the synapse. They also monitor the amount of neurotransmitter acting on other parts of the neuron as well.

In view of their role, autoreceptors become an interesting object of speculation when contemplating the future of drug abuse. Is it possible to develop a drug that would "trick" these autoreceptors? Could such a drug manipulate these receptors into thinking that more transmitter should be released when in fact that were not the case? Would it not be possible to combine this new drug with cocaine to produce an experience of pleasure that was more intense and perhaps more prolonged than the pleasure obtained with cocaine alone?

As you might have guessed from the existence of autoreceptors, one of the big questions in this area concerns the relationship between the type of receptor and its location. It is an area fraught with ambiguities. D-1 and D-2 receptors are known to be located on the postsynaptic membrane. Both types are activated by the neurotransmitter as it conveys a message from the presynaptic neuron.

Both receptors are found on the presynaptic neuron as well. Given this complexity, the questions are obvious. Which receptors, and in what locations, are the most heavily involved in the effects of cocaine? While the most appealing candidate is the D-2 postsynaptic receptor, this cannot be known with certainly until receptor classification is more precise, and until more is known about their varying functional roles. For example, is it the case that the functions of a given receptor type change from a presynaptic to a postsynaptic location?

Finally, the changes that receptors show when they undergo prolonged drug stimulation are of equal import for the future. Receptors are not static components of the membrane. They exhibit dynamic changes over time. Some types of drug treatments can render receptors more sensitive to neurotransmitter. Other drugs can make receptors less sensitive to synaptic messages. These effects are well enough known in pharmacology to have names. They are called *up-regulation* and *down-regulation,* respectively. These dynamic changes in receptor status are thought to be important in many drug actions. The beneficial effects of several drugs used in the treatment of mental illness is thought to result from their ability to produce these kinds of long-term changes in receptor status.

All of the possibilities for future drug development must be viewed in this context of changing receptor sensitivity. If there is a dopamine receptor type that is crucial for cocaine-initiated pleasure, what would be the consequences if it were up-regulated? Could down-regulation be used to diminish the intensity of the cocaine response, or perhaps to eliminate it all together?

Cocaine Receptors and Dopamine Transporters

Finally, there is the question of the cocaine receptor itself. How many are there? Where are they located? What is the nature of the relationship between drug action at the receptor and the inhibited reuptake of the neurotransmitter?

The reuptake mechanism on the dopamine neurons is called a *transporter.* It is the work of this transporter that is blocked by cocaine. The drug, acting on or near the transporter site, prevents the neuron from performing its normal function of transmitter reuptake. Thus, cocaine interferes with the neuron's ability to self-regulate.

In order to block this transport, cocaine must bind to the cell, to its receptor. Unfortunately, no one has a very good idea of just where this receptor is. In addition, several cases are known in which drugs appear to act at more than one receptor site. If there is more than one cocaine receptor, which one is related to the inhibition of neurotransmitter reuptak?

Some scientists have suggested that the cocaine receptor is the dopamine transporter itself. The transport process, the reuptake, is blocked, they suggest, because the drug is taking up the space which is normally occupied by the neurotransmitter. This view suggests that the relationship between cocaine and dopamine is more or less an accidental one. There is no special cellular mechanism set aside, so to speak, to respond to cocaine. The drug "just happens" to fit a membrane component that otherwise serves a completely natural function, that of terminating the action of the transmitter dopamine.

Others have suggested that the cocaine receptor is distinct from the dopamine transporter but that it is located adjacent to it on the membrane. This view maintains that cocaine binds to its own receptor and in the process produces a deformation in the transporter that renders the reuptake mechanism nonfunctional. In this view, a tantalizing one to say the least, there *is* a special relationship between brain cells and cocaine. Brain cells are "ready," as it were, to respond to the drug whenever it comes along. All of us, in other words, have been prepared by evolutionary processes to be sitting ducks for the cocaine molecule. We are all potential victims in waiting.

This position suggests some intriguing possibilities. It is unlikely that there is any adaptive value in responding with euphoria to the coca plant. A process of natural selection for this response is probably not the reason for the existence of the cocaine receptor. The more likely possibility is that the brain may produce its own chemicals that target this receptor. Such chemicals could function to some extent in a way analogous to cocaine. They would be naturally occuring chemicals that underlie normally occuring pleasure states. (The suggestion is not fanciful. A similar state of affairs is known to exist with respect to opiates. The brain produces its own chemicals—they are called enkephalins or endorphins—that produce opiate-like effects through their action at opiate receptors.)

Regardless of which view of the cocaine receptor is correct, the probability of obtaining increased knowledge about it may be a source of some apprehension. Consider the possibilities. Drugs produce their effects, for good or ill, as a function of their ability to activate an appropriate receptor. Having detailed knowledge about a drug receptor is analogous to having detailed knowledge about a building site upon which a house is to be constructed. The house can only be better for it. So, too, for the drug. As scientists unearth more detailed knowledge about cocaine's action in the brain, it is very likely that information will emerge concerning the cocaine receptor. This information, in turn, will allow a more precise specification of the way in which cocaine activates this receptor. The stage will thereby be set to fine-tune the drug-receptor interaction. And, remember, this interaction is likely to be precisely the one that initiates a chain of events leading to the experience of intense pleasure.

These, then, are the types of questions being actively pursued at the present time. Out of all this work is most certainly to emerge a long line of chemical probes of the brain's pleasure circuitry. Some of these drugs will be put to good use. Some may find application in the field of mental illness. Others may be found to be useful in increasing achievement levels of children with certain kinds of learning difficulties. Still others will probably find utility in areas that are now unimaginable.

What to Do When the Genie Is Out of the Bottle?

Will such future drugs be abused? Will their users appear on our streets in epidemic proportion, torturing our society even more than cocaine does today?

The answer is almost certainly yes. There has not yet been a time when the fruits of scientific discovery about pleasure-yielding drugs have not shown up on the street. All of these new *pleasure probes* will find their way into recreational use. All of them have the potential to become drugs of abuse that are more threatening to society than crack and cocaine are today.

Legitimately manufactured pleasure probes will be diverted to recreational street use in the same way that amphetamine has been. The market will exist. Entrepeneurs will supply the demand. Law enforcement efforts will be directed and redirected in a continuing but futile attempt to stem the tide. To the extent that the tide is diverted temporarily, illicit laboratories will emerge to manufacture the sought-after chemicals.

And how much worse it may be in this future beyond cocaine! Today's makers of designer drugs have precious little to work with in comparison to what they will have in this anticipated future. In the world beyond cocaine much more sophisticated knowledge about the brain's pleasure circuitry will be available. Receptors in this circuitry may be discovered that provide more direct access to the brain's centers of pleasure than cocaine and crack do today. Correspondingly, new drugs will be developed that activate these receptors with a precision now unknown. These drugs will be new keys to pleasure, new ways to unlock primitive circuits in the brain, new ways to subvert brain mechanisms that have guided evolution and selection processes throughout the millennia, new snares to entrap increasingly large numbers of young people into the wasting business of drug addiction. The future beyond cocaine may well see the apotheosis of the philosopher Thomas Hobbes's description of life as "an unending quest for pleasure after pleasure that ceaseth only in death."

Our society must undertake a drastic reformulation of the drug problem before this future becomes a reality. What is necessary is nothing less than the complete revision of some of our most cherished ways of thinking about the drug problem. Unless this is done, and soon, the future beyond cocaine does not inspire much confidence.

Chapter 9

Rethinking the Future Beyond Cocaine

Rethinking the Nature of the "Enemy"

Drugs are not mysterious. Drugs of abuse do not operate on the mind in arcane ways to produce their characteristic changes in a person's perception of himself and the world around him. Drugs are, rather, chemical agents that modify the normal patterns of biochemical operation of brain cells. Their actions in the brain and the subsequent effects that they produce are subject to rational understanding. A first step in dealing with any drug of abuse is to understand clearly what these actions are and how they produce their effects.

Until evidence accumulates to the contrary, each drug should be regarded as unique. Drugs can certainly be categorized in numerous ways, as is done routinely in science and medicine. In these situations, however, the classification is done only following the accumulation of hard evidence that supports it. Furthermore, in this endeavor drugs may be subject to classification in more than one category. Imipramine, a drug that is used to treat depression, is quite reasonably classified as an antidepressant. It could be, with equal justification, classified as a central nervous system stimulant.

The important thing is to recognize that in either case the categorization is made by knowledgeable scientists on the basis of hard evidence about all of the properties of the drug. In particular, drugs are not placed in a common category when they differ widely among themselves.

When it comes to official classification of drugs of abuse, however, little or no attention is paid to most of the important properties of the drugs that are placed in this category. These drugs are classified essentially on the basis of the likelihood that they will be abused. (Another factor, whether or not the drug has a currently recognized medical use, is also involved, but the overwhelming consideration in the classification is the abuse potential of the drug.) While most people who use drugs illegally are well aware of important differences among drugs like cocaine, marijuana, heroin, PCP and others, these differences are largely ignored by a system that classifies them simply as drugs of abuse. In most cases, the characteristics which are disregarded are those which knowledgeable scientists would consider to be the most important properties of the drugs.

To get an idea of just how wrongheaded all of this is, consider the drugs listed in Table 9.1. These drugs are grouped into a

TABLE 9.1

CLASSIFICATION OF COMMON DRUGS THAT AFFECT
THE MIND AND BEHAVIOR

Classification	Effect on Mind/Behavior	Examples of Specific Drugs
General Nervous System Stimulants	Arousal/increase in activity	Cocaine, amphetamine, methamphetamine, caffeine, nicotine
Central Nervous System Depressants	Depression/decrease in activity	Alcohol, barbiturates, Valium, Librium
Narcotic Analgesics	Pain suppression/ quieting, euphoria	Heroin, morphine, Codeine, Percodan
Drugs Used to Treat Depression	Arousal/elevation of mood	Imipramine, Desipramine
Drugs Used to Treat Schizophrenia	Varied/reduction of psychotic symptoms	Phenothiazine, Haloperidol
Hallucinogens	Varied/altered state of consciousness	Marijuana, LSD, PCP

classification system that is in common use by scientists like pharmacologists, psychiatrists and psychologists, who study and work with drugs that affect the mind and behavior. The listed drugs produce these effects, of course, because their site of action is the nervous system.

The first thing to note is that the table includes the most commonly abused drugs in our culture, including cocaine, heroin, morphine, barbiturates, amphetamine, alcohol, LSD, PCP, and marijuana.

The most important thing to notice about the table is that the drugs of abuse shown there are not all classified in the same way. Some of them are CNS stimulants, like cocaine and amphetamine. Some are CNS depressants, like alcohol and barbiturates. Others are narcotic analgesics, like heroin and morphine. Still others are classified as hallucinogens. (These are sometimes referred to as psychedelics.) The commonly abused drugs, in other words, come from almost every one of the major categories that have been established by people who know the most about drugs that affect the mind and behavior. These drugs of abuse differ among themselves in major ways.

It is worth paying some attention to this method of classification. Note in particular the varying effects on behavior represented by these drugs. Some of them, like the CNS depressants, have a subduing effect. That's why they are called, on the street, *downers*. In relatively small doses, they may have transitory activating effects, as in the case of alcohol. These effects are the result of the depressant action of the drugs on portions of the CNS, and are always followed by behavioral depression.

CNS stimulants, on the other hand, are referred to on the street as *uppers*. They lead to increases in activity level and mental alertness. Their behavioral effects are the opposite of the CNS depressants.

Narcotic analgesics like morphine are used clinically to relieve pain. Other narcotics are used to control cough and to stop diarrhea. It is of considerable significance that they produce these effects without a general depression of the CNS. The reason is that they have different sites of action than do drugs like barbiturates. While narcotics and barbiturates are both "drugs of abuse," the behavioral picture of someone taking narcotics is quite different than that shown by someone taking CNS depressants.

A similar comparison could be made among the other classes of drugs listed in the table. They are classified differently because they act at different sites in the nervous system and produce different patterns of effects on activity.

In society's approach to these drugs, however, such differences are obscured. The drugs are all classified simply drugs of abuse as a part of the Drug Problem. In contrast to the way in which informed scientists and physicians define these same drugs, the official classification pays virtually no attention to what these drugs of abuse do, or do not, have in common. The only thing they have in common, in fact, is that they have all been judged to be drugs of abuse. The drugs are radically different in chemistry, in their sites and mechanisms of action in the brain, and in the effects that they produce. All of these differences are ignored in classifying them drugs of abuse.

Lumping wildly disparate drugs into the common category of drugs of abuse is counterproductive to attempts to deal rationally with the abuse problem. The categorization freezes our thinking and reduces our freedom to act intelligently. Classification on this basis removes the room to maneuver that is necessary if the problem of drug abuse is to be approached in a rational manner. To label substances drugs of abuse and let it go at that is to say, "Don't bother me with facts. Let me deal with the problem in my own misinformed and counterproductive way."

Once a compound is classified a drug of abuse, no more intelligent thought is required to figure out how to deal with it. The drug can be dealt with like all other drugs in that category. The same moral judgements can be made. The same legislative philosophy can be applied. Educational efforts can be simplified since they all boil down to the same thing. Citizens legitimately concerned about the drug problem can be reassuringly fed the same coping strategy by those in authority whenever a new drug raises its head.

The only problem is that it doesn't work.

We should know better. The simple evidence of our own experience should tell us better. There is something manifestly absurd about a system that implies that marijuana and crack, and the problems that they pose for society, can be meaningfully discussed as a package. It flies in the face of common sense to assume that the presumed similarities between them, simply because they have both been classified drugs of abuse, render insignificant their manifold differences. Consider these important differences between the two drugs:

1. They are vastly different in addictive potential. No one, not even the most dedicated of the supporters of the current official classification scheme, would seriously maintain that it is as easy to become addicted to marijuana as it is to cocaine.
2. The consequences of abusing the two drugs are drastically different. The cocaine user is much more likely to progress to intravenous injection. This IV route of administration opens the door to a multitude of disease sequelae that are unknown in the case of marijuana.
3. The possibility of experiencing a serious medical emergency is infinitely higher with cocaine than it is with marijuana. I doubt that you will ever see a Helen in the emergency room of a hospital solely as a result of having used marijuana. Her story is common when cocaine is used.

Marijuana, to put it simply, is a safer drug than cocaine. This is an important distinction if you are really interested in devising rational drug policies. It is a distinction, however, that is most often lost when both are classified drugs of abuse.

One can only wonder if our present cocaine problem would be less acute if we had applied this kind of analysis to troublesome drugs a number of years ago, say, at the time of the Harrison Narcotic Act, when cocaine was mistakenly categorized as a narcotic.

From all of this it is possible to make an important generalization: Drugs must be dealt with on an individual basis if there is to be any chance of solving the problem of drug abuse. The differences among drugs is of greater importance to a rational drug policy than is any similarity that is presumed to exist as a result of classifying them all as drugs of abuse.

It is time to start all over in our efforts to classify drugs that have become problems for society. We must throw out the current "official" classification of drugs, throw out the DEA schedules in current use. Most such methods of classification make a rational treatment of drug problems more difficult than necessary. They do this because they preempt habits of thought. They constrain thinking and inhibit the emergence of innovative approaches to the drug problem.

Rethinking the Nature of the "Victim" of Drug Abuse

The time has come to distinguish between people who use drugs and people who abuse them: Drug use and drug abuse are not synonymous.

This notion is liable to make a number of people uncomfortable. Above all, it should disquiet many of the individuals who formulate our drug policies. The laws that have been enacted are designed to make this distinction difficult or impossible to maintain. Drugs are classified according to their abuse potential, and legal constraints make their use (and often their possession) an illicit activity. In practice, therefore, it is impossible in this system to differentiate between the mere use of drugs and their abuse.

In particular, the present system makes it very difficult to do any serious study of the relationship between drug use and drug abuse. Most of what we think we know about the factors that lead to the abuse of drugs is gathered from after-the-fact studies of people who are already well into the mire of drug problems. We study individuals who have come to the attention of the criminal justice system, the hospitals, the clinics and so on. We see them at a time when their use of the drug is out of their control. In this setting it is virtually impossible to reach any reliable conclusions about the factors in drug use that have contributed to drug abuse. This kind of information is what the scientist calls retrospective data. Such data are usually gathered in an opportunistic fashion, far from the way in which an ideal scientific study would be designed.

How much better off we would be if we were able to study drug users *before* they became drug abusers. If we were able to study them over time, systematically, in their specific cultural context, we might learn something about why some people can control their drug use, and even walk away from it, while others become more drug-dependent. We might begin to separate the factors which are involved in the use of drugs from those which predispose people to dependence on drugs. While some work like this has been done, it is difficult to accomplish much under current conditions.

At present, the use of a drug that has been classified as a drug of abuse often makes the user, by definition, an abuser of the drug. The distinction between drug use and drug abuse is lost at the outset, at least from a legal standpoint. Studying this individual over time is not an easy thing to do. He may not be very forthcoming about his behavior, since he might consider himself to be running some significant risks, like loss of job or even imprisonment. He may even object that, in asking for his participation in such a study, asking him, that is, to continue his drug use, we are encouraging him to break the law.

Some authorities will tell you, of course, that they recognize that there is a difference between using a drug and abusing it. But the system does not allow for this distinction. Of the 750,000 people arrested each year for violating the drug laws, about 75 percent are arrested for simple possession. These people can be convicted under the drug-abuse statues without any determination that they are drug abusers in any sense other than that they have broken the drug laws.

Is the distinction important? You bet it is. We make it all of the time. The distinction is invoked informally every time we say:

"Well, I know that my teenage son does a little pot every now and then, but it's nothing serious. There's a lot of peer pressure out there. I don't think he's really into drugs in a big way."

"We did a lot of weird drugs in the sixties, when I was younger. But, at some point I just kinda walked away from it."

"If you drink, don't drive. If you drive, don't drink."

The difference between the two ideas is also maintained at a more formal level. The distinction is made every time attention is drawn to the 230,000 deaths annually that are associated with tobacco, in a country where the government has for years subsidized the growing of the toxic plant. The distinction is made every time a law is used to convict someone of drunk driving because his blood alcohol level exceeded legally permissible amounts.

The distinction is workable and is regularly recognized in our culture for some drugs (e.g., alcohol and tobacco) but not for others. In the case of alcohol, the distinction is so important that the one attempt made in this country to abolish it was abandoned as being unworkable. It caused more harm than good. The attempt was called the Noble Experiment, or National Prohibition. The repeal of this misguided constitutional amendment thirteen years after it was enacted was a frank recognition that it was in the best interests of society to distinguish between the use of a drug and the abuse of a drug.

Drug abuse should be regarded as a *medical* condition that results from *excessive* drug use that leads to adverse consequences for the person and those around him. Drug abuse should not be defined as the one-time or occasional use of a drug unless it has been shown that this pattern of use does, indeed, produce these adverse consequences. We support the distinction in the case of alcohol and tobacco, but that is nothing other than a traditional, unreasoning prejudice in favor of some drugs and not others.

It is important to distinguish between these two ideas because doing so promotes a better understanding of the reasons why people use drugs. It helps in seeing that the factors that lead people to drug use are not necessarily the same as those that lead to drug abuse. It leads to the recognition that drug use arises from social and environmental forces of the kind that shape and mold all our behavior. The demands and pressures of living require that we develop means for coping with stress. Some of us develop nondrug strategies, whereas others find relief in illegal drugs. Many of us develop a mix of solutions, where nondrug strategems are mingled with the use of varying amounts of legal drugs, including alcohol, nicotine and prescription medications like Valium.

Additional considerations enter the picture when the individual moves from drug use to drug abuse. After all, given any reasonable distinction between drug use and drug abuse, the vast majority of us are drug users (either legal or illegal) while very few of us, relatively speaking, ever become drug abusers. To become a drug abuser requires the operation of factors in addition to those that predispose us to the simple use of drugs.

Feeling Good Sometimes vs. Never Feeling Good at All

It is easy to list some of the reasons why people use drugs: peer pressure, curiosity, rebellion, feelings of anxiety and insecurity. All of these, and more, are well-recognized factors that push people toward drug use.

On the other hand, a lot of drug use occurs in situations where these factors do not seem to play a role. People use drugs in the absence of obvious peer pressure. Similarly, a good deal of time can be spent in taking a drug that the person knows well, where his curiosity has long since been satisfied. Drug use may likewise persist long after rebellion has run its course, and large amounts of drugs are taken in situations where anxiety is a stranger and security is well established.

There is a reason for this lack of perfect relationship between these factors and drug use. All "causes" of drug use such as these are what might be called *proximal* causes. They operate in the foreground. These factors come into play in a close time relationship with the use of drugs. They enact their role when all the players are on the stage. They do not do a lot to explain drug use in any fundamental sense, because they can equally be invoked to explain a number of other human activities that do not involve drugs. Peer pressure and anxiety, for example, can motivate a range of activities from defeated withdrawal to strong striving toward achievement, none of which has any connection with drug use. In this situation, the suspicion grows that there are more distal, or fundamental wellsprings involved in drug use. It further seems likely that, given the pervasive nature of drug use, such a distal cause would aid in seeing the distinction between drug use and drug abuse.

One such fundamental factor has to do with states of consciousness. All of us, at more or less regular intervals, search for things to do that distract us from the day-to-day business of living. Some of us jog, some read, others go fishing, still others go to church, and so on. All of these things, and many other activities like meditation, prayer or listening to music, serve to distract us from our daily troubles and sources of worry. Activities like these take us outside of ourselves, however briefly, and withdraw our attention from "the human condition."

This is not a trivial matter. Homo sapiens seem to have an intrinsic need for periodic alterations in his conscious awareness of himself and his surroundings. Such mental gear-shifting is probably essential, or at least conducive, to his survival. Periodic respite from the demands of the workaday world probably renders us more able to cope with it when the rest interval ends. There is a considerable amount of shared cultural wisdom on this point, and some of it is taught more or less directly to each generation as it comes along. All work and no play, after all, does seem to make Jack a dull boy.

Drugs are without peer when it comes to producing changes in awareness. Have a couple of beers; smoke some marijuana; take a hit of cocaine. See how your troubles melt away. See how rapidly and how well your worldview changes. This is awareness alteration with a vengeance. Drugs do this so well, in fact, that the truly remarkable thing is that most of us are *not* thoroughly benumbed by drugs most of the time.

Drugs like cocaine excel at producing altered states of awareness because of their ability to tap into the basic biology of the brain. The response is quick and intense. It is unlikely that any of the other consciousness-altering ploys that we have devised can transport us so rapidly and completely from a humdrum daily existence to a plane where the pain is less hurtful and life is more tolerable.

In rethinking the nature of the victim, it is a good idea to keep this pervasive characteristic—this periodic need to alter awareness—firmly in mind. It suggests that we are, in fact, prone to drug use simply because of what we are. Most of us have a powerful need to "get out of ourselves" or to "stand back from the situation" from time to time. Drugs are one of the ways we have discovered to accomplish this.

It is necessary to concede that drugs have a potential "claim" on humans, simply because they are human. Drugs have exerted this claim for thousands of years. References to the use of drugs to yield pleasure are as old as recorded history. The opium poppy is described as just such a vehicle in the ancient Babylonian texts from the time of Hammurabi, about 3000 B.C.

Why should this be the case? There are several ways to answer this question. At the level of brain organization, the answers seem fairly clear. The preceding pages have pointed out that drugs like cocaine are "naturally" satisfying to humans because they are able to call into action brain mechanisms related to survival. The activation of pleasure circuits in the brain guarantees that drug taking will be rewarding. People will in general respond favorably to a drug experience because of the way in which their brains are organized. At this level, the satisfaction associated with drug taking can be regarded as a fortuitous outcome of having a brain well structured to increase the survival of the species.

The important factor under consideration here is that the drug user must be understood as a biological creature. Acknowledgment must be accorded to his phylogenetic roots, to the evolutionary history that makes him so responsive to the pleasure produced by drugs.

There is another level of analysis that is equally important. Most of us do not take drugs constantly. And why not? There is a sense in which the answer to this question may speak volumes to an understanding of those who use drugs to excess. Several lines of thought suggest themselves.

To begin with, it may be that most of us understand that the downside potential is too great. We know that the great euphoria, the great temporary release from care and anxiety that drugs can provide, does not come free. There is addiction; there is expense; there is disease; there is the possibility of imprisonment. There are a lot of undesirable consequences that we associate with drug-induced feelings of well-being. They may loom large in our consciousness and argue forcefully against our becoming seriously involved with chemical alteration of our mental state.

On the other hand, the very immediacy of the pleasure supplied by cocaine, and the certainty of its occurrence, suggests that another factor might be operating here. It may be that those people who do not become compulsive drug users have a superior ability to resist the temptation of immediate gratification. They are able to forego, as the compulsive drug user cannot, the immediate high, the instant euphoria, offered by drugs, in favor of more lasting satisfactions. This ability to resist the temptation may appear in various dress. Perhaps one's religious beliefs militate against defiling God's temple with foreign substances. Or drug use may be seen as a hindrance to getting a job or to advancing in it. Fear of arrest and imprisonment may make the forswearing of drugs the easier thing to do. Doubt over the inability to control one's own impulses can serve to keep an individual from becoming involved with powerfully rewarding drugs. And so on.

This proposition, while simple, is potentially revolutionary in the context of a rational drug policy. Think about it again. Given the biological readiness to respond intensely to pleasure-giving drugs, the wonder is that *all* of the population is not more or less continually involved with such compounds. In looking for reasons for compulsive drug use, it may be more important to understand why most of us don't engage in such behavior than it is to understand why a minority of our number do self-destruct in this way.

Thinking along these lines changes the nature of the battle. Rather than engaging our efforts in a war against drugs, it directs our attention to the nature of the drug user. Instead of focusing our attention on the drug abuser as an evildoer, it leads us to consider the drug abuser as an individual who has been victimized by his biology. Most important, it suggests that it is not inevitable that this person be a victim, not inevitable that he be held captive by his biological inheritance. After all, most people in our society are able to resist the lure of constant and immediate gratification offered by drugs. Drawing on their example, we are led to hope that others can be shown how to resist the snares that drugs place in their path.

We are not entering uncharted waters here. This matter of choosing between immediate and delayed gratification has been studied for years by psychologists. This is not too surprising, since our ability to live together in social harmony depends on the acquired ability of most members of the group to delay gratification of their needs and desires. The process goes by several names. Political scientists call it the *social contract*. Freud described it as the process whereby the child is taught to repress basic aspects of his biological inheritance so that the social group is not ripped asunder by the unbridled search for immediate gratification. The fact that civilization has, by and large, been able to maintain itself for thousands of years is strong evidence that such social contracts work.

The process occurs so pervasively and in so many guises that we are often unaware that it is going on. Child rearing can be thought of as the process by which an older individual continually teaches a younger person to postpone immediate gratification in order to attain a "better" reward in the future. Managing money, saving for a rainy day, doing unto others (now) as you would have them do unto you (later)—much of what is called the socialization process takes this form.

The question really revolves around why the process "takes" better in some situations, in some people, than in others. As you might expect, no one knows for sure. But there are some things that seem to be essential to acquiring the ability to postpone gratification:

- A sense of personal security.
- A feeling that tomorrow will be better than today.
- A conviction that your efforts to better yourself will bear fruit.
- A feeling of personal worth.
- A confidence that "the system" will not betray your decision to forego immediate pleasure.

When these things are lacking, it may well be that one's existence is just as Hobbes described it when he said, "Life is solitary, poor, nasty, brutish and short."

These feelings and convictions are basic to the taming of biological imperatives like pleasure-seeking, which must be controlled if individuals are to live successfully in social groups. They are easy to state. Knowing how to bring them about in any individual case is another matter. But surely it is worth trying to find out. For, in the final analysis, one thing is certain. When large numbers of people do not experience the safety and the hope that are embodied in the feelings listed above, their need for periodic alterations of consciousness will be intensified. They will also be readily receptive to the numbing of their condition that is available in the form of drugs like cocaine.

Rethinking the Consequences of Drug Use: The Question of Gains and Losses for Society

Everyone knows what the consequences of out-of-control drug use are—lost productivity, broken homes, ruined lives, disturbed relations with foreign governments. There are only losses, no gains.

But a rethinking of the potential costs associated with current programs aimed at reducing drug abuse leads to some frightening possibilities. These costs include:

1. A severe reduction in domestic tranquility and safety. Out-of-control drug use has spawned an out-of-control cycle of crime and violence that has fundamentally altered the way our citizens view life. Street crime, muggings, murders and armed robbery are perpetrated on our citizens to a degree that seems to signal the

breakdown of law and order. Our streets have become the battleground of warring armies. Highly armed, rival drug cartels contend for control of the lucrative cocaine trade. They kill one another ruthlessly, and they often, in the process, kill innocent bystanders, as well. As this process has escalated, more Americans in some areas of our cities are afraid to venture out of their homes. This is an intolerable cost in "the land of the free and the home of the brave."

2.   Grossly inflated budgets for law enforcement and prisons. The only obvious result thus far of the heating up of the War on Drugs has been an enormous increase in the cost of fighting it. These costs are borne by each and every taxpayer. The war requires a diversion of resources to pay the bill. The costs continue to escalate with no sign at all that the war is even possible to win. Victory in selected battles is announced from time to time. But even those who have fought in them, the law enforcement personnel, suffer no illusions that they are winning the war.

3.   The threatened loss of cherished civil liberties. Forced and involuntary drug testing looms as a frontal assault on basic constitutional guarantees that American citizens have enjoyed since the founding of the republic.

And this may be only the beginning. The threat of drugs can be used as a way to rationalize almost any abridgment of civil liberties. Some years ago attacks were made on the right of American citizens to be safe in their homes. The "no-knock" proposals of that period would have allowed police to enter and conduct searches of homes without having to bother with a search warrant—only, of course, if the police had a suspicion that drugs could be found there.

4.   Computers make the drug-engendered threat to civil liberties even more threatening. Big Brother really is watching. In some states, if your doctor prescribes a narcotic to ease the pain that you are suffering following a surgical operation, your name and the drug prescribed are entered into government computers. This, of course, is part of the War on Drugs, too. Never mind that narcotics obtained by ordinary citizens in this fashion contribute negligibly to the drug problems of the country.

Why, then, is this done? For several reasons. First, it is possible—the existing computer technology makes it easy. Of more importance, however, is the persistent lure of catchphrases and simplistic solutions. The reasoning goes like this: heroin and other narcotics are drugs of abuse; drugs like Percodan (a physician-prescribed drug) are narcotics; hence, if we are to control narcotics, we had better keep up with Percodan use, even that prescribed by physicians. After all, if we have to create a dossier on everyone in the country, detailing the most private aspects of his or her life, it will be a small price to pay for ridding the nation of the sourge of drugs.

Rethinking Treatment and Rehabilitation

The only long-term solution is education. Educational efforts have, of course, been a part of our approach to the drug problem, but they have not been markedly successful. If education is said to be the answer, it is necessary to examine why previous educational efforts have met with such limited success.

When it comes to problems with drugs, we have never understood the nature of the educational task that was called for. We have never grasped the basic idea that, if education is to be successful, it must begin with an enlightened assessment of why drugs are such an attraction. Instead, the approach has been to present drugs as inherently evil substances, on the same plane with popular conceptions of the devil. In fact, the theological analogy is appropriate. Drugs are evil and those who take them are evil. Drug abusers may be regarded as morally corrupt individuals who have traded their souls for the fleeting pleasure afforded by drugs.

The educational efforts, if they can be called that, that have stemmed from this type of simplistic world view have relied on two basic strategies. The first is *fear*. The notion is that you can keep people from taking drugs by making them so afraid of the consequences that they will recoil in horror from the very idea of drugs. There are various ways of eliciting this fear.

1.   Raise the possibility of severe legal repercussions—jail time, big fines—if your drug use comes to the attention of the authorities.

2.   Graphically depict the alleged biological effects of drug use. Tell young people that their brains will be fried by drugs. Tell them that drugs may lead them to kill themselves or to kill someone else.

3.   Tell young people that their genetic material will be damaged by drugs. Make them aware that drug use may injure their chromo-

somes or increase the likelihood that they will father or give birth to deformed children.

These and numerous variations on the theme of fear have been one of the major vehicles that have carried the antidrug message. The other is what might be called The Know-Nothing, Blissful-Ignorance approach. The idea here is to round up several well-known public figures, usually professional athletes, who are assumed to be idolized by young people. These figures are then trotted out in convenient forums, usually brief ads on TV, to proclaim their message. In essence, the message is, "If you want to be like me, *just say no.*" In this appeal there is not much attention paid to *why* you should just say no. The idea is that if the prestige of the speaker is high enough he can get his audience to follow him blindly, with no questions asked.

There is no evidence that either of these strategies has had an appreciable positive effect. In view of what we now know about cocaine, this is not surprising. Both strategies ignore the fundamental relationship that exists between the drug and the biology of the drug taker. They fail to understand that this relationship is so strong and deeply ingrained that the worst possible strategy is to ignore it or to deny that it exists.

People do not take drugs because they are wicked. They do not take drugs because they are perverse. They take drugs because the drugs make them feel good. Very good.

Any meaningful program of drug education must begin with an acknowledgment of this fact. While it may seem contradictory and self-defeating, it will be necessary to begin attempts to educate people by admitting frankly that some drugs can make them feel really good about themselves. This is especially true when it comes to educating young people. You do not begin with fear or with role models. You begin with solid, accurate information. You tell people the truth.

Most people will know if you are not telling them the whole story. They will see immediately that you have something to hide. The bottom line is that there is no reason to hide anything. Most people already know that drugs produce good feelings. By avoiding this obviously relevant piece of information, you will lose credibility. This is especially devastating when your audience is young people. They already are predisposed to be suspicious of the preaching of their elders. The task is to gain their confidence and respect, not to alienate them further. At worst, you will appear to be lying to them. Their own experience and the experience of their friends have provided them with a lot of information on the way drugs make you feel. Best to begin by acknowledging the obvious and proceed with your credibility intact.

There is no room in a drug education program, no matter what the target audience is, for anything other than solid, factual information about drugs. If you want people to hear you when you tell them about the downside of drug taking, you will have to be right up front about the short-term, good feelings that drugs produce. Do not begin the message at the end, with the doom-and-gloom observations of the real havoc that unwise drug use can bring. Begin at the beginning, where the audience is, with the acknowledgement that drugs do, in fact, produce effects that most people regard as pleasurable. The idea in the educational effort, as revolutionary as that may seem, is to keep your audience with you. You want them convinced that you know what you are talking about and that you have something important to say. You do not want to be tuned out prematurely. Education does not take place when no one is listening.

Our educational efforts should go something like this:

"You bet. I know. Drugs like cocaine and crack can give you a real high. There's no doubt about it. Let's talk about some of the ways the drug makes you feel, and let's try to understand what the drug does in your body to make you feel that way. There's really nothing magic about this process and you ought to know all that you can about it.

"The problem is that getting high in this way can have some bad consequences. These don't happen all of the time, but they happen in enough cases that I want you to be aware of them. You owe it to yourself to be informed about the way the drug produces these undesirable effects, just as it was a good idea to see how the drug brings about the more pleasurable feelings.

"The important message in all of this is that drugs are chemicals that are uniquely able to modify some fundamental aspects of the way your brain works. Drugs are able to tap into some of the most basic aspects of what it means to be a human being. In some cases, these drug-induced changes in the way your brain works can be so profound that they can come to dominate your life. They do this because they can exploit brain mechanisms related to biological survival at the most basic level. In doing this, they can cause other important aspects of your life, aspects other than survival and feeling good, to become less and less meaningful to you. Unfortunately, among the things that are most apt to recede in importance are those personal characteristics that we think of as uniquely human—your ability to love and to care for other people."

In the final analysis, people will use drugs responsibly only when they see that it is in their own best interest to do so. Responsible drug use includes not using drugs at all. It implies, in addition, an appreciation that some drugs are potentially more devastating than others. There is a corollary to this: educational programs that really do lead to responsible drug use might very well find people steering away from drugs like cocaine—steering themselves away, that is, because they have been led to see that it is in their own best interest to do so. Our history of drug control efforts offers stark testimony to the fact that the tactics of fear fail miserably in appealing to this self-interest. Programs that attempt to profit from the persuasive power of cultural heroes, in the absence of meaningful intellectual content, are equally nonproductive.

The drug problem is solvable. The fact that we have not yet managed a solution says more about our intelligence and inventiveness than it does about the difficult nature of drugs themselves. For almost a century we have been following policies that have failed miserably while remaining essentially unchanged. This persistent infatuation with narrowly conceived programs that are based upon a studied ignorance of useful scientific data is one of the more remarkable follies of recent human history.

One wonders what our great-grandchildren will think of our efforts. What will they do in the years beyond cocaine? Based upon our own experience and predilections, a pessimist would anticipate that they will perpetuate the errors that we have bequeathed them, that their policies will be our policies, that they will still be fighting the war that we were unable to win.

But possibly, just possibly, they may be smarter than we are. One hopes that they will be able to stand back and pose rational questions, that they will ask knowledgeable people for hard data about the drugs that pose problems in their world. One hopes that they will not be so attached to proposed solutions, simply because they have proposed them, that they will lose the flexibility required to come to terms with a complex world.

It is within our power to make it easier for them. By rethinking the problems that cocaine has forced upon us, we may be able to devise strategies that are effective in reducing the ravages of out-of-control drug use. We may be able to bequeath to our great-grandchildren a world in which drugs are not the scourge that they are today. Rather than passing on to them the legacy of failure which has fallen to us, perhaps we will find the intelligence, the creativity and the will to leave them programs that work.

Index

A

Absorption, 65-66
Acquired ability, reward centers, 78
Addiction, 25-26, 31, 67, 72, 82, 102
Adulteration, 42
AIDS, 41, 105-106, 111-112
Alcohol, 43, 145, 146
Alkaloid, 38
Altered message transmission, 88-90
Altitude, 37-38
Alzheimer's disease, 88
Amphetamines, 30, 145, 146
  and brain sensors, 13
  cottage industry of, 122-124
Anesthetic drugs, 24, 56
  altered message transmission, 89
  cocaine substitutes, 130-131
Antibiotics, 64
Anxiety, 62, 152
Aphrodisiac, 23, 53, 56, 57
Arousal level, changes in, 50-51
Aschenbrandt, Theodor, 22
Auditory hallucinations, 58
Autonomic nervous system (ANS),
    61, 62
Autoreceptors, 139-140
Awareness, altered states of, 152-153

B

Bacteria, 64
Baking soda, 44
Barbiturates, 145, 146

Behavioral changes, 49, 145
Blissful-ignorance approach, 159
Blood-brain relationship, 43
Bloodstream, function of, 64-67
Bodily sensations, 49, 52
Body temperature, 63
Brain,
  center activation, 76-79
  chemical structures, 129
  evolution of, 79-82
  functions of, 3
  impact of drugs, 13-15, 42-43, 54-55
  limbic system, 134
  localization of function, 73-74
  pleasure circuits, 96-97, 101,
        133-135
    and receptors, 137-140
    survival mechanisms, 153-154
  rat study, 68-72
  reward centers, 69-72
  selective message transmission, 88
  snorting impact, 42-43
  stimulating effects on, 63
Broca's speech area, 73-74

C

Caffeine, 38, 145
Cardiovascular system, 62-63
Cash crops, 115
Central nervous system,
  cocaine and, 54-55, 63-64
  depressants, 145-146
  and information flows, 84-88

Chemical formulas, 124-126
Chemical messages, 91-95
Chewing process, 20, 37-38, 40
Civil rights, and war on drugs, 33,
    35-36, 119, 157-158
Classification of drugs, 145-149
Coca plant, 19
    components of, 37-38
    as form of social control, 18-20
    Indian legends of, 19-20
    military applications, 22
    use in medications and tonics,
        21-23
Coca-Cola, 26-27
Cocaine, 145, 146
    behavioral responses to, 49
    blockade of presynaptic reuptake,
        99-103
    fever, 63
    forms of, 42-46
    from plant to drug, 21-22
    hydrochloride, 40
    narcotic classification, 30, 145-146
    parties, 7
    population use, 15, 104-105
    problem, scope of, 104-120
    psychosis, 23, 57-59
    purification process, 38-40
    solutions to, 11, 160-162
    subversion of biochemical control
        centers, 82-83
    unique aspects of, 12-16
Codeine, 145
Coercion, as prevention, 113-114
Coffee bean, 38
Colombia, and coca plants, 116
Compulsive drug use, reasons for,
    154-155
Computers, 157-158
Conquistadores, 18-19
Consciousness, states of, 152-153
Context, and cocaine use, 49
Control, restoration of, 3-4, 5-6
Cost-benefit analysis, 104-112. *See
    also* Hidden costs
Cottage industry, amphetamines,
    121-126
Crack, 39-40, 44-46, 147-148

D

Dehumanization, cost of, 109-110
Delusions, 58-59
Demand,
    costs to reduce, 117
    disruption of, 34-35
Depression, drug treatment of, 96
Designer drugs, 124-126, 128-132
Desipramine, 145
Disorders of movement, 87-88
Distillation, 43
Dopamine,
    receptors,
        chemical formula of, 124
        and pleasure centers, 97-103
        types of, 136-138
    transporters and cocaine receptors,
        140-142
Down-regulation, 140
Downers, 146
Doyle, Sir Arthur Conan, 27
Dr. Jekyll and Mr. Hyde (Stevenson),
    28
Drugs,
    action, 60-64
    catchwords, 9-10
    chemical structure, and specificity,
        90
    classification problems, 145-149
    and depression, 145-146
    difference of, 10-11
    future modifications, 132-143
    receptor, 99-103
    and schizophrenia, 145-146
    serendipity findings, 127-128
    testing of, 35-36, 118-119
    use and abuse, distinctions of,
        36-37, 149-158

E

Education, 35, 158-162
Electrical probe study, rats, 68-72
Emergency room 1-4
Energy level, 49, 50-51
Enzymes, 94
Equanil, 128

Erection, 56
Ergot, 128
Erythromycin, 64
Erythroxylon coca, 19
Ether, 44
Experience, and brain events, 74-75
Extraction process, 38-40

F

Fear,
    and antidrug message, 158-159
    physical effects of, 60-61
Feelings, and cocaine use, 46-48, 6-9,
        62. *See also* Pleasure centers
Fermentation, 43
Fight or flight response, 60-61
Fleischl, Ernest, von, 23, 57
Foreign policy, 32-33, 36, 115-117
Formication, 59
Free-base cocaine, 39-40, 44-45,
        66-67
Freud, Sigmund, 22-24, 47-48

G

Gaedecke, Freidrich, 21
General nervous system stimulants,
        effects of, 145-146
Genitals, cocaine application, 56
Grand mal seizure, 3-4
Gratification, immediate and
        postpone, 154-156
Greed, and designer drugs, 131
Gums, 40-41

H

Hallucinogens, effects of, 58-59,
        145-146
Haloperidol, 145
Halstead, William, 24-25
Harrison Narcotic Act, 30
Helen,
    cocaine reaction, 5, 6-7, 8
    emergency room admittance, 1-4
    personality of, 1
Hemp plant, 38

Heroin, 145, 146
    and brain sensors, 13
    morphine derivative, 43-44
Hidden costs, war on drugs, 107-112,
        115-119
Hofmann, Albert, 128
Huntington's disease, 87
Hypodermic syringe, 43

I

I Get a Kick Out of You (Porter), 29
Imipramine, 144-145
Indians, and cocaine use, 18-20, 37-38
Information flows, central nervous
        system, 84-91
Inner-city youth, and values, 110
Interdiction, 115-117
Intravenous injection (IV), 41, 45,
        50-51
Isolation of cocaine from coca plant,
        21-22, 38-39, 42

J

James, William, 85
Johns Hopkins Medical School, 25

K

Know-nothing approach, 159
Koller, Carl, 24

L

L-dopa, 90, 95, 97
Larmarck, Jean-Baptiste de, 19, 20
Law enforcement, 30, 34, 114-115,
        117-118, 156-157
Legislation, prohibition of cocaine, 29
Librium, 127, 145
Lidocaine, 130-131
Limbic system, 134
Liver, detoxification organ, 41
LSD (lysergic acid diethylamide), 124,
        125, 128, 146

M

Mariani, Angelo, 21
Marijuana, 38, 115-116, 124, 145, 147-148
Meaning, and the nervous system, 85-86
Medial forebrain bundle, 136
Medicine, and coca plant, 21-23
Memory, effects of cocaine, 3-4
Meprobamate, 128
Message termination, 98
Message transmission, 88-89, 91-95
Methamphetamine, 124, 145
Military, and coca plant, 22
Monardes, Nicolas, 20
Mood, 49, 51-52
Morphine,
    effects of, 24, 26, 145, 146
    isolation process, 43-44
    and Naloxone, 102
Multiple receptors, 138
Multiple sclerosis, 87

N

Naloxone, 102
Narcotic analgesics, effects of, 145-146
Natural form of cocaine, 44
Nervous center, information flow, 84-91
Neural energy, 86-87
Neurons, 76-77, 136
    communication function, 83-88
    interference with communication transmission, 88-91
    and synaptic transmission, 91-95
Neuroscience, 128-129
Neurotransmitters, 92-97, 136, 140
Nicotine, 145
Niemann, Albert, 21
Nigrostriatal pathway, 90
Novocaine, 26, 130-131
Nucleus accumbens, 134-136

O

Olds, James, 68-73, 101
Opiate narcotics, drug specificity, 89-90

Opiate receptors, 95, 102
Opium,
    cash crops, 115-116
    and morphine, 43-44
The Opium War, 26
Organized crime, 32
Orgasm, 56, 75
Overstimulation, prevention of, 94-95

P

Parasympathetic nervous system (PNS), 61
Parke-Davis Pharmaceutical Company, 29
Parkinsonism, 87, 90, 97
PCP, 145, 146
Peer pressure, 152
Penicillin, 64
Perception of pleasure, 75
Percodan, 145
Peru, 17-20
PET scans, 77
Phenothiazine, 128, 145
Physical changes, 46, 48
Pizarro, Francisco, 17-18
Pleasure, 81
    centers, 13-14, 16, 81-83, 101
        circuitry, 96-97, 133-136, 137-140, 153-154
        dopamine-secreting neurons, 97-98
    chemistry of, 97-99
    connection, 68-73
    temporal aspects of, 135
Police, dehumanization of, 109-110
Porter, Cole, 29
Postsynaptic neuron, 91-96, 139-140
Presynaptic,
    neuron, 91-96, 139-140, 102, 136.
        See also Dopamine receptors
    reuptake, 98
Price of success, 107-108
Prohibition, 30, 151
Proximal causes, 152
Psychosis, 23, 57-59
Public confidence, cost to, 109
Public health, costs to, 111-112
Pure Food and Drug Act (1907), 27
Purification process, 38-40

R

Rats, electrical probe study, 68-72, 81
Receptors,
    changes by chemical stimulation,
        139-140
    decoding the environment, 85-86,
        97, 99-102
    types of, 137-140
Recreational users, 40-41
Rehabilitation, rethinking of, 158-162
Retarded orgasm, 56
Reuptake process, 99-102
Reward centers, 70-72, 76-79, 82, 101
Ring compounds, 127
Roche Labs, 127
Royalty, commodity use of coca plant,
        19-20

S

Schizophrenia, drug treatment of, 96
Self-image, changes in, 48-49
Sensory stimulation, 55, 77
Sexual response, 52-57, 74-75
Sign of Four (Doyle), 27-28
Snorting, 40-41, 42-43, 50-51, 66
Social constraints, loosening of, 57
Social contract, 155
Social control, biological nature of
        man, 113-114
Social rewards, 81
Spanish explorations, 17-19
Speech center, 73
Speed Labs, 123-124
Spinal cord injury, 75
Sternbach, L.H., 127
Stevenson, Robert Louis, 28
Stimulant drug, effects of, 22, 63-64
Stimulation, and pleasure, 69-72
Stroke, 73
Substitute drugs, 26

Success, costs of, 114-120
Supply, disruption of, 34-35, 36
Survival, and pleasure centers, 82
Sympathetic nervous system, 60-62
Sympathomimetic drug, 61
Synaptic messages, 91-95, 140

T

Tactile hallucinations, 58
THC, 38
Thorndike, E.L., 81
Tonics, 26-27
Transduction, 87
Transporters, 140-142
Treatment, rethinking of, 158-162
Tuberculosis, 28

U

University of Cracow, 127
Uppers, 146
Upregulation, 140
Urine testing, 35-36, 118-119

V

Valium, 127, 145
Values, inner-city youth, 110
Vasoconstrictor, 66
Ventral tegmental area (VTA), 98, 136
Victim,
    costs, 108
    new concepts of, 149-156
Vin Mariani, 21

W

War on drugs,
    hidden costs, 108-112, 114-120
    potential costs, 156-158
Wine, 21

ABOUT THE AUTHOR

John C. Flynn, Ph.D., is a professor at Baylor University in Waco, Texas, where he teaches psychology and neuroscience. He has also done extensive teaching in the areas of psychopharmacology and drugs and behavior and has written articles for leading scientific publications.